# LIFE-THREATENING PROBLEMS IN THE EMERGENCY ROOM

Problems in Anaesthesia

This book is dedicated to Alan Millward and Tilman Riemanschneider

# LIFE-THREATENING PROBLEMS IN THE EMERGENCY ROOM

## Problems in Anaesthesia

### Anne J Sutcliffe

BSc, MB, ChB, FFARCS, ARPS

*Consultant Anaesthetist,*
*Birmingham Accident Hospital,*
*Birmingham, UK*

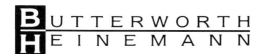

Butterworth-Heinemann Ltd
Linacre House, Jordan Hill, Oxford OX2 8DP

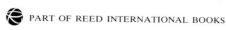 PART OF REED INTERNATIONAL BOOKS

OXFORD LONDON BOSTON
MUNICH NEW DELHI SINGAPORE SYDNEY
TOKYO TORONTO WELLINGTON

First published 1992

**British Library Cataloguing in Publication Data**
Sutcliffe, Anne J.
  Life-threatening Problems in the
  Emergency Room. – (Problems in
  Anaesthesia Series)
  I. Title   II. Series
  617.9
ISBN 0 7506 0370 4

Set 10 on 11 point Times by
TecSet Ltd, Wallington, Surrey

Printed in Great Britain at the University Press, Cambridge

# Contents

Contents

Contents

Contents

## Contents

# *Preface*

In a hospital, the Accident and Emergency (A&E) department can be one of the most interesting and exciting areas to work. The patients have a variety of illnesses and injuries ranging from trivial to life threatening. Doctors working in the A&E department have the challenge of being the first to diagnose and treat the patient and, if all goes well, the satisfaction of initiating the path to an uncomplicated and speedy recovery.

The A&E department can also be a frightening place to work. Severely ill and injured patients often arrive with little or no warning. They may present with a variety of bewildering symptoms and signs. Senior colleagues may not be instantly available. The doctors receiving the patient must have the confidence and competence to commence prompt and effective life-saving treatment.

Recent reforms in the National Health Service have placed more and more emphasis on the quality of care given to patients. Quality of care has many facets. At one end of the spectrum, it is expected that all hospitals provide hotel services of an acceptable standard. At the other end of the spectrum, doctors are expected to make accurate diagnoses and to provide prompt and effective treatment which will result in a speedy recovery with minimal complications. Whatever aspect of the quality of care is considered, true quality can only be achieved by tailoring the care provided to the individual patient's needs.

Many A&E departments have a set of protocols for the treatment of individual diseases and injuries. Advanced Trauma Life Support and Advanced Cardiac Life Support courses are organized in many areas and provide national treatment protocols. There can be no doubt that the use of protocols is preferable to a poorly planned, and possibly unsafe, approach to the management of patients. Of necessity, however, protocols are rigid. In a crisis they can be life saving but they do not permit deviations from the protocol to suit the particular needs of an individual patient. In an ideal world, all doctors would be able to diagnose all conditions and to provide effective treatment. Unfortunately, the world is not, and is unlikely ever to be, ideal. In the A&E department, protocols will continue to be used. Nevertheless, improvements in care should be possible, particularly if a pathophysiological approach to patient management is adopted. In spite of the diverse causes of illness and injury, the life-threatening pathophysiological derangements encountered in the A&E department are limited in number. It is not unreasonable to suggest that doctors working in A&E should familiarize themselves with the recognition of these pathophysiological changes and to strive to understand the mechanisms involved and corrective measures needed for treatment in an attempt to achieve the best possible outcome following disease or injury. The object of all medical interventions is to return the patient to the community in the best possible physical condition, in the shortest possible time with the least possible disruption to his life.

This book is a companion to *Problems in Anaesthesia*. Like its predecessor, it aims to stimulate a rational approach to the management of patients in the A&E department based on pathophysiological principles. It is written primarily for anaesthetists. Increasingly, however, there is an overlap between the role of anaesthetists and the role of A&E specialists and for some groups of patients, such as those with major trauma, a team approach to management has been adopted and proved successful. In the future, it is probable that the team approach in the A&E department will be developed still further to include the management of severely ill medical and surgical patients. This book covers problems traditionally encountered by trainee anaesthetists in the A&E department and is intended mainly for trainee anaesthetists. Senior anaesthetists may also find it helpful for teaching purposes. It also contains information of interest to A&E doctors, nurses and other paramedical staff. A common approach to problems by all members of the A&E team could lead to greater cooperation and understanding, and ultimately to an improvement in the quality of care offered to patients.

# Introduction

Patients presenting to the A&E department are notable for the variety of complaints from which they suffer. As the name of the department suggests, patients fall into two broad categories; those who have had an accident and those who have developed an acute medical or surgical condition requiring emergency treatment. In spite of the variety of presenting conditions, the pathophysiological derangement caused by a given condition and the approach to the management of that condition is often similar to that of another condition which, at first sight, may seem totally different.

A common approach to the management of all patients can be particularly helpful. There are five phases of management:

1. *Primary survey* to assess the adequacy of the airway, breathing and circulation and to diagnose life-threatening hypoxia, hypovolaemia and myocardial failure.
2. *Life saving resuscitation* to ensure airway patency and security, adequate ventilation of the lungs, restoration of circulating blood volume, support for the failing myocardium and, ultimately, adequate tissue oxygenation.
3. *Secondary survey* to establish the definitive diagnosis or diagnoses.
4. *Definitive management* appropriate to the diagnoses made in the secondary survey.
5. *Reassessment* to confirm that the patient's clinical progress matches that expected for the diagnoses made and the treatment already given and, if necessary, to modify the diagnosis and/or the treatment.

This book is divided into four parts, covering major trauma, burns, medical and surgical emergencies and specific problems relating to the management of the paediatric patient which are not covered in preceding parts. Each part covers the theoretical and practical aspects of the pathophysiological derangements suffered by each group of patients. The similarities of pathophysiological derangement suffered by different groups of patients has already been noted. In order to avoid persistent repetition in subsequent sections, there is extensive cross-referencing so that the reader can easily find the information relevant to a problem of particular interest. At first, the frequency of cross referencing may be irritating. As the layout of the book becomes familiar to the reader, it should serve to highlight the factors which are common to severely ill and injured patients who are admitted to the A&E department.

Although each part or topic can be read on its own, it is recommended that the book should be read from cover to cover on at least one occasion. The similarities of the problems presented by each group of patients will be better understood. It should be possible to apply lessons learned from one patient's problems to another patient with a different diagnosis but similar pathophysiological abnormalities. The author makes no apology for the frequent stress laid on the importance of recognizing and treating hypoxia, hypovolaemia and myocardial failure with the ultimate goal of preventing or reversing tissue hypoxia.

*Don't panic!* However urgent the situation, panicking will not help. Always remember the following principles and there will be time to think and worry about other problems later.

1. Patients die from hypoxia, hypovolaemia and myocardial failure.
2. Always check the airway, breathing and circulation first.
3. If any of these are inadequate, start basic life-saving measures immediately. If necessary, ask another person to call for the assistance of senior colleagues.
4. When the airway, breathing and circulation are secure, stand back and take your time to perform a thorough examination of the patient.
5. Define the problems and treat appropriately.

6. Monitor the patient closely, re-examine the patient at least once and assess whether the response to treatment is adequate and appropriate for the injuries or disease already identified.

# PART ONE

# Life-threatening problems of major injuries

# Theoretical aspects

## *Hypoxia, hypovolaemia and myocardial failure*

The problems which threaten the lives of all patients with major trauma are airway obstruction, difficulty with breathing and circulatory collapse. Every doctor is trained in the recognition and treatment of these problems. It is, therefore, alarming that as recently as 1988 a retrospective study of one thousand deaths from major trauma showed that at least one third of the patients who reached hospital alive subsequently died unnecessarily. Analysis of these deaths revealed that the patients had a variety of injuries which were either not diagnosed, mis-diagnosed or diagnosed correctly but treated inadequately. Trainee anaesthetists and A&E specialists may, quite rightly, believe that the diagnosis of some life-threatening injuries is beyond their present, or indeed their future, competence. This attitude perhaps explains why there were so many preventable deaths from major trauma. Using the aforementioned report as part of its evidence, The Royal College of Surgeons Working Party on 'The Management of Patients with Major Trauma' recommended that Major Trauma Centres be established where seriously injured patients could be treated by teams of senior medical staff experienced in their care. It will take time to establish Trauma Centres and even when they are established there is no guarantee that every seriously injured patient will be admitted directly to one of these Centres. Furthermore, any doctor working in an A&E department may, in the event of a major disaster, find himself treating seriously injured patients. An approach other than that based on the definitive diagnosis of injuries is, therefore, required.

In approximately 80% of the patients in whom death was considered preventable, further analysis shows that these deaths were caused by injuries which result in hypoxia and/or cardiovascular insufficiency. This suggests that a pathophysiological approach to the resuscitation of the injured is a reasonable alternative form of management; at least in the first crucial minutes after admission.

## FURTHER READING

Anderson, I.D., Woodford, M., de Dombat, T. and Irving, M. (1988). A retrospective survey of 1000 deaths from injury in England and Wales. *Br. Med. J.*, **296**, 1305–1308.

Commission on the Provision of Surgical Services. (1988). *Report on the Management of Patients with Major Injuries.* London: Royal College of Surgeons.

# The pathophysiological effects of injury

Prompt treatment of the pathophysiological, life-threatening effects of injury can be enormously helpful in preventing not only early, but also late, death after injury. Early death from injury is almost always due to hypoxia and hypovolaemia, either alone or in combination. The only exception to this rule is death due to extensive primary brain injury which affects the brain stem. Even in this case, damage to the brain stem disrupts the function of the respiratory and cardiovascular control centres causing secondary hypoxia and circulatory failure. Loss of protective airway reflexes and pulmonary inhalation of gastric contents may also cause severe hypoxia in head injured patients. Even if the primary brain injury is not severe, secondary brain damage due to hypoxia and hypovolaemia can transform a non-fatal brain injury into a fatal one. Perhaps worse, recovery without neurological deficit may be reduced to recovery with a significant neurological deficit; a situation which may, for the patient, be worse than death.

Whatever the anatomical location of the injury, hypoxia and cardiovascular insufficiency have one ultimate effect. This effect is cellular hypoxia. Cellular dysfunction occurs in the presence of primary hypoxia when anaerobic sources of energy fail to maintain energy production at the minimum level required by various metabolic processes. The severity of cellular dysfunction is not uniform amongst all organs. Skeletal muscle cells, for example, can recover normal function after 30 minutes of total ischaemia. Isolated hepatocytes can withstand two and a half hours of ischaemia but brain cells suffer permanent damage after only six minutes of hypoxia. Furthermore, in some organs such as the liver and brain, cells which are furthest away from oxygen-rich blood are more susceptible to hypoxic damage than cells which are close to the capillary network.

The cellular effects of hypoxia are, therefore, variable. In the presence of severe, prolonged hypoxia, all cells are at risk of irreversible damage. The mechanisms of irreversible damage are not completely understood. In most instances there is probably more than one mechanism involved which may include the development of cellular acidosis, the loss of adenine nucleotides from the cell, the generation of toxic metabolites such as oxygen-free radicals and tumour necrosis factor, changes in the intracellular concentration of calcium and degradation of membrane phospholipids.

Severe hypovolaemia reduces blood flow to the tissues. Inevitably, the oxygen supply to the tissues is also reduced and tissue hypoxia occurs. The results are the same as those described for primary cellular hypoxia. In addition, hypovolaemia causes ischaemia of the intestinal mucosa which enhances transfer of intestinal bacteria and endotoxins to the portal, and thence to the systemic circulation. Once in the systemic circulation, the endotoxins are capable of causing widespread damage to the capillary basement endothelium. Tissue oedema develops and causes extensive organ dysfunction.

The clinical manifestation of cellular dysfunction and death is organ failure. The adult respiratory distress syndrome, in which pulmonary oedema develops in the presence of normal left atrial pressures, has long been recognized as a late complication of a variety of insults which include injury, major haemorrhage, and sepsis. The adult respiratory distress syndrome was originally thought to be an isolated condition affecting the lungs. It is now recognized as the pulmonary manifestation of multiple organ failure. There are two reasons for delayed death after injury. The first is severe head injury with massive destruction of brain cells and uncontrollable cerebral swelling. The second is multiple organ failure. There is a large body of evidence which indicates that mortality increases in proportion to the number of organ failures and that the severity and number of organ failures is proportional to the severity of prior hypoxic and hypovolaemic insults.

Fat embolism syndrome is a condition which occurs almost exclusively after long bone and pelvic fractures. The mechanisms which lead to the development of the fat embolism syndrome are not well understood but, whatever the primary mechanism, the pathophysiological changes of fat embolism syndrome bear a remarkable similarity to those seen in the adult respiratory distress syndrome and multiple organ failure. Although fat embolism syndrome can develop in an adequately resuscitated patient who has never been shocked, there is good evidence that its incidence is increased in patients who have suffered an episode of hypoxia and/or cardiovascular insufficiency. It is likely that in patients with long bone fractures who subsequently develop fat embolism syndrome, hypoxia and hypovolaemia represent a significant secondary insult which certainly delays recovery and may reduce the quality of the ultimate outcome.

Although shock is recognized clinically by the presence of tachycardia, hypotension and intense vasoconstriction sufficient to cause a decrease in urine output, it is difficult to define in quantitative terms. The best qualitative definition of shock currently available is 'a reduction in cardiac output, and hence tissue perfusion, sufficient to cause cellular hypoxia'. The previous discussion has demonstrated the importance of hypoxia and cardiovascular insufficiency as short- and long-term causes of morbidity and death after major injury. Bedside measures of the oxygenation of individual tissues are not yet available. It is possible to obtain a global estimate of tissue oxygenation using a pulmonary artery flotation catheter to measure oxygen flux but this technique is not always appropriate in the severely injured patient when basic life-saving measures must take priority over sophisticated monitoring techniques. It is also possible to measure blood lactate levels which rise in proportion to the severity of tissue hypoxia. The results are not usually available during resuscitation and, if raised, indicate that a large oxygen debt already exists and perhaps that resuscitation has been inadequate. It is the goal of resuscitation to prevent such an oxygen debt occurring.

In order to prevent, or at least minimize, the effects of hypoxia and hypovolaemia, the clinician must be skilled in basic diagnostic techniques and have a good understanding of the physiological processes which normally maintain adequate tissue oxygenation.

## FURTHER READING

Gutierrez, G. (1991). Cellular energy metabolism during hypoxia. *Crit. Care Med.*, **19**, 619–626.

Fink, M.P. (1991). Gastrointestinal mucosal injury in experimental models of shock, trauma and sepsis. *Crit. Care Med.*, **19**, 627–641.

Westaby, S. (1988). Mediators in acute lung injury: the whole body inflammatory response hypothesis. In *Shock and the Adult Respiratory Distress Syndrome* (Kox, W. and Bihari, D., eds). London: Springer-Verlag, pp. 33–41.

Benumof, J.L., ed. (1988). Management of patients with multisystem organ failure. *Anesthesiol. Clin. N. Amer.*, **6** (1). Philadelphia: W.B. Saunders Co.

Peltier, L.F. (1984). Fat embolism. *Clin. Orthopaed. Rel. Res.*, **187**, 3–17.

# *Mechanisms for the maintenance of cellular oxygenation and some reasons for failure*

There are numerous factors which control the amount of oxygen which is ultimately available for utilization by an individual cell. All are intimately related and manipulation of one factor may adversely affect another.

**Inhaled oxygen concentration**. Under normal conditions, the inhalation of room air is sufficient to support adequate cellular oxygenation. The oxygen utilized by the cells is transported to the tissues by the red cells. If the patient is grossly hypoxic or the red cell volume has been depleted by haemorrhage or chronic anaemia, the cells may utilize oxygen which is dissolved in the plasma. The amount of dissolved oxygen can be increased by increasing the inspired oxygen concentration. It is helpful to administer 100% oxygen to all severely injured patients during resuscitation.

Fears are sometimes expressed that oxygen is toxic to the lungs. It is true that if a person with normal lungs inhales high concentrations of oxygen for more than 24 hours, lung damage can occur. There have never been any reports of lung damage caused by inhalation of 100% oxygen during resuscitation. This is probably because the period of administration is short because estimation of blood gases will permit the inspired oxygen concentration to be reduced to a more appropriate level as soon as the patient has been stabilized.

Another problem, which sometimes causes concern, is the risk of depressing hypoxic respiratory drive in the patient with chronic bronchitis. These patients are normally hypoxic and can be severely damaged by additional hypoxic insults resulting from injury. In every case, additional oxygen is beneficial. On the very rare occasions when the hypoxic pulmonary drive is depressed by supplemental oxygen, this should be rapidly detected by routine monitoring of the adequacy of breathing and can easily be treated by reducing the concentration of inspired oxygen. In the A&E department, the potential benefits of giving high inspired concentrations of oxygen to all injured patients far outweigh the potential dangers to a tiny minority.

**Transfer of oxygen to the trachea and bronchial tree.** There is no point administering high concentrations of oxygen to the patient if the upper airway is obstructed. Upper airway obstruction has many causes (Table 1.1.1). These must be promptly recognized and treated. Adequate respiratory excursion is necessary for mass transport of gases to the trachea and lower airways. Hypoxia, secondary to poor respiratory excursion may be due to inadequate cerebral control, cervical spine injury, pain in the chest wall, severe structural damage to the chest wall or diaphragmatic splinting by massive intra-abdominal haemorrhage. Rarely, major tears of the trachea, bronchi and major bronchioles can result in

**Table 1.1.1 Causes of upper airway obstruction following injury**

1.  Loss of protective airway reflexes
    (a) head injury
    (b) hypoxia
    (c) hypovolaemia
    (d) alcohol or drugs

2.  Swelling of the larynx or oropharynx

3.  Laryngeal injury or transection of the upper trachea

4.  Foreign bodies
    (a) solid food
    (b) blood clot
    (c) false teeth
    (d) knives or sharp instruments
    (e) other miscellaneous objects

massive leaks of oxygen into the pleural cavities and mediastinum and hence inadequate flow to the lower airways.

**Transfer of oxygen from the bronchial tree to the alveolar capillary membrane**. Having traversed the terminal bronchioles, oxygen must reach the alveolar-capillary membrane. This will not occur if the alveoli are collapsed due to external pressure such as pneumothorax, haemothorax or migration of abdominal contents into the chest cavity through a diaphragmatic rupture. Alveoli also collapse if air is absorbed distal to obstruction of the larger airways by inhaled solid vomitus, blood or foreign bodies. The alveolar membrane itself may be obliterated by liquids such as blood and stomach contents. Pulmonary oedema caused by fluid overload, myocardial failure or severe head injury may also impair gas transfer to the alveoli. Far more common than major airway injury is alveolar disruption due to direct pulmonary injury which should be suspected in all patients with fractured ribs, a fractured sternum or severe chest wall pain in the absence of fractures. Alveolar damage may also occur because of blast injury to the lungs or crush injury to the chest. Inhalation of acidic gastric contents damages alveoli and is a secondary insult which should, if possible, be prevented.

**Transfer of oxygen across the alveolar-capillary membrane to the blood**. Transfer of oxygen across the alveolar-capillary membrane may be restricted by damage to either or both parts of the membrane. Furthermore interstitial oedema due to fluid overload, cardiac failure or pulmonary trauma widens the distance across which oxygen must pass and impairs diffusion. Most patients with upper and/or lower airway abnormalities are hypoxic and benefit not only from definitive treatment, but also from a high inspired oxygen concentration delivered, if necessary, through an endotracheal tube.

In addition to adequate ventilation, adequate oxygenation of the blood depends on adequate perfusion of the lungs by the pulmonary circulation. If perfusion exceeds ventilation, hypoxia occurs. To a certain extent, the mismatch of perfusion and ventilation is mitigated by hypoxic pulmonary vasoconstriction and an increase in respiratory rate. Pulmonary perfusion is reduced in the presence of absolute hypovolaemia, relative hypovolaemia and myocardial insufficiency. In the injured patient, reduced pulmonary blood flow is nearly always associated with reduced systemic blood flow and, hence, reduced tissue perfusion. Factors influencing tissue perfusion are discussed in the next section. In the normovolaemic patient with good myocardial function, pulmonary capillary blood flow may also be reduced by the presence of fat globules, microemboli from blood products and microthrombi which form on damaged capillary membranes.

Most oxygen is transported to the tissues bound to haemoglobin and a reduction in erythrocyte numbers can cause tissue hypoxia. Anaemia is thought to cause global tissue hypoxia if the haemoglobin concentration falls below 7 g/dl. In the normal person, a fall in haemoglobin to 7 g/dl would only occur if 50% of the blood volume was lost and was not replaced by erythrocyte containing blood products. Lesser degrees of anaemia may, however, cause regional tissue hypoxia, the severity of which is increased by concomitant reductions in tissue blood flow.

**Circulation of blood to the tissues**. In order for oxygen-carrying erythrocytes to reach the tissues, there must be sufficient blood flow. This depends on there being an adequate circulating blood volume. There may be an absolute diminution in blood volume in injured patients due to haemorrhage or a relative reduction in volume due to vasodilatation as a result of spinal cord injury or alcoholic intoxication. A reduction of blood volume also occurs due to sequestration of oedema fluid in injured tissues. There are numerous neural and humoral compensatory mechanisms which cause vasoconstriction in an attempt to match the circulating blood volume to the vascular space. Initially vasoconstriction occurs in 'non-essential' tissues such as the skin, muscle and gastrointestinal tract. A blood volume deficit of greater than one litre causes pre- and post-glomerular vasoconstriction in the kidneys and renal blood flow and glomerular filtration rate are reduced by 30% and 50% respectively. Losses of greater than 1750 ml result in a reduction in glomerular filtration rate to less than 20% of normal. Eventually, if fluid replacement is not started, blood flow to the brain and heart is reduced to critical levels.

In order to ensure blood flow to the tissues, adequate myocardial muscle contractility is equally as important as an adequate blood volume. In response to hypovolaemia, the heart rate will normally increase. This response may be obtunded in patients with pre-existing heart disease or myocardial contusion. Extrinsic compression of the heart by blood or air may cause tamponade and reduce cardiac output. A tension pneumothorax may distort the major veins thus impeding venous return and reducing cardiac output. Air embolism is very rarely a cause of reduced cardiac output in injured patients. Severe brain injury is also an uncommon cause of a poor cardiac output. Inadequate tissue oxygenation leads to anaerobic metabolism and lactate production. Myocardial contractility is reduced by severe metabolic acidosis but, in the injured patient, this is rarely the only cause for inadequate myocardial contractility.

It is quite common for injured patients to be mildly hypothermic on admission to hospital. Their temperature can drop still further during examination and resuscitation. This may be because clothes have been removed to facilitate examination or cold fluids are administered rapidly. Severe hypothermia reduces cardiac output. The transit time through capillaries is decreased in low flow states and by an increased haematocrit which can occur when resuscitation is achieved primarily with concentrated red cells. Blood viscosity, and hence transit time, also increase as body temperature falls.

**Transfer of oxygen from the capillaries to the tissues**. Microemboli are found in the tissues of all injured patients with fractures and other severe injuries. Some of these microemboli arise from the bone marrow and fatty tissues. Others may be the debris from transfused blood. Capillary membranes are also damaged by toxic metabolites released from injured tissues and thrombi are deposited in areas of damage. Whatever the reason for the occurrence of microemboli and thrombi, there is no doubt that they block the capillaries and impede blood flow to the tissues.

The affinity of red cells for oxygen is increased by a metabolic alkalosis which can be caused by over zealous treatment of a metabolic acidosis with sodium bicarbonate or by the use of controlled mechanical ventilation with greater than necessary minute volumes. Similarly, hypothermia increases the affinity of haemoglobin for oxygen. In all these instances, less oxygen is released to the tissues. Finally, toxic metabolites such as complement, arachidonic acid metabolites, and free oxygen radicals, which are released after injury and shock, interfere with mitochondrial oxygen utilization.

**FURTHER READING**

Snyder, J.V. (1987). *Oxygen Transport in the Critically Ill.* Chicago: Year Book Medical Publications.
Bernstein, D.P. (1991). Oxygen transport and utilization in trauma. In *Trauma Anesthesia and Intensive Care* (Capan, L.M., Miller, S.M. and Turndorf, H., eds.). Philadelphia: J.B. Lippincott Company, pp. 115–165.

# *Treatment goals*

Hypoxia and hypovolaemia are the two physiological states which pose the greatest threat to life in the severely injured patient. Both cause tissue hypoxia, the disruption of cellular function and, ultimately, cell death. The physiological mechanisms by which cells are oxygenated are complex. It is possible for the A&E anaesthetist to manipulate many of these mechanisms to facilitate tissue oxygenation. In the process of manipulating one aspect of oxygen transport, it is possible to inhibit another aspect of transport. In order, to treat the patient effectively the anaesthetist must always bear in mind the ultimate goal of treatment which is to restore tissue oxygenation to normal. The following guidelines for therapy may be useful:

1. Ensure adequate oxygenation and ventilation of the respiratory tract.
2. Restore the circulating blood volume to normal.
3. Optimize myocardial contractility.
4. Optimize arterial red cell content to facilitate oxygen transport and capillary blood flow.
5. Normalize erythrocyte oxygen affinity.

Practical aspects

# *Ethical considerations*

Most patients suffering major injuries are, prior to their accident, young, healthy and fit. With the exception of brain, spinal cord and eye injuries where cell regeneration cannot occur and reconstructive surgery is not possible, most injuries are capable of healing with minimal or absent residual disability. The outlook for many injured patients admitted to the A&E department is, therefore, excellent.

Patients with severe head injuries and spinal cord injury present a difficult problem because the quality of survival may be poor. In the case of severe head injury, it is not yet possible to predict the outcome with any degree of certainty. Furthermore, the outcome may be worsened if there are any delays in the treatment of hypoxia and hypovolaemia. Similarly, although the level of spinal cord injury can be estimated with reasonable accuracy, oedema may raise the level temporarily by one or more dermatomes, minor bony movement may render partial lesions reversibly complete if the problem is recognized and promptly treated, and hypoxia and hypovolaemia can cause greater permanent damage if not promptly treated. Thus, there is little scope or need for making ethical decisions about the treatment of severely injured patients. Prompt aggressive treatment is essential in all instances. Ethical decisions, such as the treatment of pneumonia in severely handicapped patients, are not relevant to the A&E department.

In general, elderly patients do less well than their younger counterparts with identical injuries. The data concerning outcome relating to severe injury and age have yet to be collected in quantities which allow irrefutable predictions regarding outcome to be made. Initially all patients, regardless of age, should have life-saving resuscitation commenced promptly. When the secondary survey has been completed, the age and medical problems of the patient are known, and the patient's prognosis has been discussed with the relatives, there may be a case for deciding that certain conditions such as renal failure should not be aggressively treated. It may be appropriate for these problems to be discussed while the patient is still in the A&E department but it is unlikely that irrevocable decisions will need to be made. Departmental guidelines may be helpful but ultimately, with due regard to the constellation of problems relevant to that particular patient, the decision will be made by senior doctors, the patient if his mental state permits it and the patient's relatives. Of necessity, the guidelines may be restricted to delineating the patients in whom treatment *may* be inappropriate, the type of treatment which *may* be inappropriate, the grade of doctor who should in collaboration with the patient and his relatives make these decisions, and, finally, whether such a decision should ever be made in the A&E department.

# The causes and diagnosis of upper airway obstruction

There are many causes for upper airway obstruction. These are listed in Table 1.1.1 (page 13). It is not necessary to make a definitive diagnosis in order to treat upper airway obstruction. It is sufficient to recognize one or more of the following clinical signs.

**Assess the verbal response to questioning**. Before touching any patient, it is customary for the doctor to introduce himself. This introduction is normally followed by some pleasantry such as 'how are you?', 'what happened to you?' or 'what is your name?'. In addition to being common courtesy and perhaps providing specific clinical information, this questioning will also help to assess the state of the upper airway. An appropriate verbal response from the patient indicates that he is conscious, the airway is patent and ventilation is intact. An inappropriate response indicates an altered level of consciousness which may be accompanied by airway incompetence. Mild hypoxia causes anxiety and verbosity. Severe hypoxia, head injury, alcohol or drug abuse can cause a reduction in conscious level such that the verbal response is inappropriate, incomprehensible or absent.

**Look for injuries to the upper airway or signs of abnormal affect**. Obvious injuries to the scalp, facial soft tissue or facial skeleton, bleeding from the nose or mouth and external wounds to the neck are clues that there may be upper airway obstruction. The abusive or uncooperative patient may be merely drunk, but this diagnosis should not be assumed until other, remediable causes of hypoxia have been ruled out.

**Listen for abnormal respiratory sounds**. Snoring, gurgling or gargling sounds may indicate partial pharyngeal obstruction. Wet sounds indicate the presence of saliva, blood or stomach contents in the pharynx and that the patient is at risk of pulmonary inhalation. Inspiratory stridor indicates narrowing of the airway at laryngeal or glottic level and may be due to a foreign body or laryngeal swelling. Hoarseness is rare, but if it occurs suggests the diagnosis of laryngeal fracture.

**Feel for air on expiration**. Its absence, in the presence of respiratory effort, is a certain sign of upper airway obstruction.

**Smell the expired air**. Alcohol on the breath may indicate intoxication which in combination with other causes of unconsciousness may obtund reflex control of the airway and place the patient at risk of pulmonary aspiration.

**Look for cyanosis**. Cyanosis does not occur unless there is at least 5 g/dl of deoxyhaemoglobin in the circulation. It is, therefore, only present if hypoxia is severe. Long before clinical cyanosis is apparent, other signs of upper airway obstruction should leave the anaesthetist in no doubt that some form of airway management is essential. The use of a pulse oximeter will show decreased oxygen saturation before cyanosis is apparent and is a monitoring device which can be quickly attached to the patient on, or even prior to, admission to hospital.

**Look for the use of accessory muscles of respiration**. In his efforts to breathe through an obstructed upper airway, the patient may use the accessory muscles of respiration. Flaring of the nostrils, tracheal tug, intercostal recession and the use of abdominal muscles are all clinical signs of excessive respiratory effort which may be a reflection of upper airway obstruction.

# Pitfalls in the diagnosis of upper airway obstruction

**Hypoxia from other causes**. Injury or obstruction to the lower airways also causes hypoxia. Signs of hypoxia such as anxiety, confusion, uncooperativeness, reduced oxygen saturation of the blood or cyanosis do not necessarily indicate an upper airway obstruction. If, however, there are other clinical findings which suggest upper airway obstruction, such as obvious upper airway injury, noisy respiration, head injury, or massive blood loss sufficient to obtund protective airway reflexes, the patency of the upper airway must be secured.

**Chest wall or pulmonary injury**. These injuries, or pain subsequent to them, may cause difficulty in breathing, hypoxia and the use of the accessory muscles of respiration. These signs can mimic upper airway obstruction. External signs of injury to the relevant parts, palpation of the chest wall to detect asymmetry of movement, painful rib fractures or subcutaneous emphysema, auscultation of the lungs for areas of decreased air entry, crepitations or bronchospasm and radiological examination of the chest may clarify the diagnosis. If there is any doubt, the upper airway should be secured.

**Cervical or thoracic spinal cord injury**. Injury to the thoracic spinal cord or the lower cervical spinal cord will paralyse the intercostal nerves and hence abolish intercostal muscle activity but diaphragmatic function is preserved because the phrenic nerve is intact. In the absence of normal intercostal muscle function, the excursion of the diaphragm becomes more obvious and the accessory muscles may be used to assist with respiration. This type of injury may mimic upper airway obstruction particularly if hypoxia causes a decrease in conscious level.

22

**Multiple injuries**. The differential diagnosis of upper airway obstruction can be tricky. Diagnosis may be even more difficult in the presence of two or more injuries which cause the same clinical signs. Some examples include concomitant head and chest injuries, head and cervical spine injuries or chest and abdominal injuries with severe blood loss leading to loss of consciousness. If there is any doubt about the patency or security of the upper airway, endotracheal intubation is indicated.

# General management principles for upper airway obstruction

**If in doubt, secure the airway**. To the experienced clinician, the diagnosis of upper airway obstruction should not be a problem. The inexperienced clinician may find the diagnosis less easy. If there is any doubt about the patency of the airway or the adequacy of protective airway reflexes, it should be secured before the breathing and circulation are assessed and, if necessary, treated.

**Cervical spine fracture or dislocation**. The possible presence of a cervical or thoracic spinal cord injury with neurological deficit has already been mentioned. The clinician should never forget that the cervical spine can be fractured or dislocated without neurological deficit. In this situation, hyperextension or hyperflexion of the neck will cause movement of the cervical vertebrae and possibly irrepairable damage to the cervical spinal cord. Until a cervical spine fracture or dislocation has been excluded, all airway manipulations should be performed without moving the neck. Cervical rigidity can be maintained by the use of a rigid cervical collar, sandbags placed on either side of the neck to prevent rotation and taping the head to a spinal board to prevent extension or flexion, or by maintaining manual in-line traction of the neck by a third party with experience of the technique. If the patient regurgitates or vomits, there is a risk that stomach contents will be aspirated into the lungs. The team caring for the patient must be aware of this possibility and be prepared to 'log roll' the patient onto his side. Management of the patient with actual or potential spinal cord injury is discussed further on pp. 33 – 34.

# Methods of airway control

There are many methods of controlling the airway. The method chosen will depend on the reason that control has been lost, the expected duration of the loss, the advantages and disadvantages of the technique, the expertise of the doctors treating the patient and complicating factors such as the risk of aspiration of stomach contents or the presence of a cervical spine injury. Careful consideration of the potential problems and constant practise of the techniques on anaesthetized patients is the key to successful management of the airway in the A&E department. The following discussion considers the range of techniques available. In certain situations, some have clear advantages. Complications are described in some detail because in situations where more than one technique is applicable, the risk of complications may be the deciding factor. When making decisions, the anaesthetist should never forget that prolonged hypoxia is more dangerous than most of the common complications associated with the techniques used for airway control. The airway must be secured rapidly. As a general rule the simplest, least invasive technique which fulfils all the requirements for complete airway control should be chosen. Fear of potential, but rare, complications should not be allowed to override the prime objective of airway management which is to ensure that there is a clear passage for oxygen to enter the lungs and that the lungs are protected from acid stomach contents and blood.

**Suction**. The upper airway may be obstructed by blood clot, foreign bodies or solid vomitus. Removal of the clot, foreign body or food may occasionally be sufficient to clear the airway, as may suctioning of liquid vomitus from the oropharynx. More commonly, continued bleeding or excess salivation is an ongoing problem which compounds poor airway control due to other causes. The most important of these causes is unconsciousness due to head injury. The airway is compromised because in the unconscious patient the tongue falls backwards into the oropharynx and there is a risk of pulmonary inhalation because the laryngeal reflexes are depressed. Suction may be sufficient to remove saliva or blood but does not guarantee a safe airway unless other measures are also taken.

**Removal of foreign bodies**. Rarely, the sole cause of upper airway obstruction is the presence of a foreign body impacted above or in the larynx. The commonest foreign bodies are solid food, false teeth and chewing gum but the anaesthetist should be prepared for surprises. If the patient is cooperative, the offending object may successfully be removed with forceps. If this is not possible the patient may require a temporary tracheostomy while the foreign body is removed surgically. Very rarely the upper airway is obstructed by a knife or other sharp instrument. It is imperative that this is not removed until the effects of removal, such as haemorrhage or airway obstruction, have been considered and prepared for. Again, a temporary tracheostomy may prove to be the safest method of airway control in anticipation of removal of the knife and subsequent corrective surgery.

**Manual methods of airway control**. In recent years, the training of ambulance personnel in the techniques of airway control has become increasingly sophisticated. Furthermore, medical flying squads, or doctors of pre-hospital care groups such as the British Association of Immediate Care, are attending the scene of major accidents more frequently. It is, therefore, rare for patients to reach hospital with poor airway control due solely to temporary hypoxia or untreated hypovolaemia. The anaesthetist should, however, remember that this situation may arise. The administration of oxygen and fluid combined with manual control of the airway for a few minutes may be all that is required for airway control to be re-established and protective airway reflexes to recover. The chin lift, in which the mandible is lifted upwards, is the simplest and safest method of manual airway control because the neck is not extended. An alternative method is the jaw thrust. In this case, the mandible is lifted not only upwards, but also forward. Airway control by either method may be improved by the use of an oropharyngeal or nasopharyngeal airway. An oropharyngeal airway is difficult to insert if the patient's jaw is clenched and may provoke coughing or vomiting. This problem is not unusual, even in the patient with obtunded airway reflexes. The nasopharyngeal airway may be easier to insert and is usually better tolerated by the patient. No matter how easy the nasopharyngeal airway is to insert, there is always a risk that bleeding will occur.

**Oesophageal obturator airway**.  This type of airway is a blunt, cuffed tube which is inserted into the oesophagus. The inflated cuff is supposed to seal the oesophagus. The tube is fenestrated in the part which lies in the oropharynx and is attached to a face mask which, if correctly applied, forms a seal. The device can be used to ventilate the lungs but is inefficient. There is also a high incidence of regurgitation because of the poor seal provided by the oesophageal cuff. Developments from the oesophageal obturator airway, such as the oesophageal gastric tube airway, have not proved to be any safer or more effective.

**Laryngeal mask airway**.  The laryngeal mask airway is a newer airway adjunct. It is an effective method of airway control in the unconscious patient if there are no other causes of obstruction such as foreign bodies or laryngeal swelling. The inflated cuff lies in the oropharynx and provides a relatively effective seal which permits ventilation of the lungs. There is still some doubt about the ability of the cuff to protect the lower airway of the unconscious patient who vomits or regurgitates. For this reason, it is probably not wise to use a laryngeal mask airway in the patient with a full stomach unless there is a compelling reason to do so. The laryngeal mask airway could, however, be life saving if the patient is hypoxic, intubation has failed and a cricothyroidotomy or tracheostomy will take time to perform.

The laryngeal mask airway can be used as an aid to oral endotracheal intubation. Local or general anaesthesia is necessary if the airway reflexes are active. Having positioned the laryngeal mask, a gum elastic bougie is threaded through the mask into the trachea. After removal of the mask the endotracheal tube is passed over the bougie into the trachea. A similar technique has been described to aid fibreoptic intubation. Both techniques are time consuming but worthy of consideration for difficult cases.

**Orotracheal intubation**.   Endotracheal intubation will guarantee patency of the upper airway and will protect the lower airway if the reflexes are obtunded. Orotracheal intubation is the technique with which anaesthetists are most familiar. It is most easily performed if the head is raised on a pillow and the neck is extended a little. This should never be contemplated in the unconscious patient until a cervical spine injury has been excluded. If a cervical spine injury is suspected, intubation should always be performed with an assistant to maintain cervical in-line traction. In the A&E department, therefore, orotracheal intubation may not be as easy as in the anaesthetized patient. Intubation may also be made more difficult by major facial injuries or bleeding into the oropharynx. As has already been mentioned, unconscious patients may still clench their jaws. Furthermore, airway reflexes may be obtunded but not sufficiently to permit intubation without the risk of causing vomiting or coughing. Sometimes, intravenous general anaesthesia may be required before intubation can be safely achieved. This too can be difficult, because muscle relaxants should never be used unless the ability to secure the airway is certain. Inhalational techniques or local anaesthesia can be considered. Both take time and, for different reasons, may be difficult in the presence of copious saliva or blood. Both cause loss of the protective airway reflexes prior to optimal intubating conditions being obtained so the patient is at risk of pulmonary inhalation until the endotracheal tube is passed and the cuff is inflated. Thus, although most anaesthetists probably prefer the oral route for endotracheal intubation, the technique does have its problems.

**Nasotracheal intubation**. Some doctors recommend blind nasal tracheal intubation for the unconscious, but spontaneously breathing, patient who may have a cervical spine injury. This is because it should be possible to intubate the patient without flexing or extending the neck. The technique is, however, associated with a number of problems.

Unless the anaesthetist is skilled in the technique of nasotracheal intubation, vomiting, coughing, bleeding from the nose, laryngospasm and hypoxia be provoked. Most patients with loss of airway control and a potential cervical spine injury are head injured. All the complications listed aggravate the primary brain injury or have the potential to increase intracranial pressure. Nasotracheal intubation is easiest to perform on awake patients because muscle tone is maintained in the tongue. Local rather than general anaesthesia is preferable because tone in the tongue is maintained but,. even if local anaesthesia is used, tone may still be minimal if the patient is unconscious because of his injuries. There may be problems with achieving adequate local anaesthesia in the presence of bleeding or excessive salivation because the anaesthetic solution becomes diluted. If intubation is urgent, there will not be time to administer an antisialogogue. Another limitation to the technique of blind nasal intubation is that the patient must be breathing as the breath sounds are used to guide the tube into the larynx.

Nasal endotracheal intubation under direct vision is associated with all the problems described for the oral route, whether or not the patient is breathing. Furthermore, in the presence of a cribriform plate fracture, the nasotracheal tube could pass into the skull and introduce infection or cause direct injury to the brain.

**Cricothyroidotomy (minitracheostomy).** Intubation of the trachea through the cricothyroid membrane can be life saving if the airway is obstructed at or above laryngeal level. Several commercial kits are available and with a little practice, the technique is easy to perform. In the moribund patient, anaesthesia is unnecessary. Otherwise, infiltration of the skin with local anaesthetic is all that is required. It is essential to ensure that the trachea is incised in the midline and that the tube is situated in the trachea. Most commercially available minitracheostomy tubes are 6 mm or less in internal diameter. They are only suitable for short-term relief of the totally obstructed airway in the spontaneously breathing patients because the small internal diameter of the tube causes significant resistance to ventilation. They can also be used for short periods to ventilate apnoeic patients. Minitracheostomy tubes are uncuffed and do not provide protection against pulmonary aspiration of stomach contents.

All anaesthetists should be capable of performing a minitracheostomy. There may be a problem if the cricothyroid membrane is difficult to palpate because of swelling or obesity. As an alternative, a large bore needle can be used to puncture the membrane. Ideally a cannula of at least 2 mm internal diameter should be used. It is almost impossible to breathe through such a narrow cannula but ventilation using high flows of oxygen is possible although carbon dioxide clearance is suboptimal. If the patient is in extremis, even insufflation of oxygen is worthwhile.

Complications from cricothyroidotomy are not common. Sometimes, if the puncture is not in the midline, bleeding occurs. If the anatomy is grossly distorted, puncture of the major blood vessels in the neck is possible. It is also possible to insert the cannula or tube into the soft tissues of the neck. It is vital to ensure that the cannula is correctly positioned and air can be freely aspirated before ventilation is commenced, particularly if high gas flows and pressures are being used. It is also theoretically possible for the posterior wall of the trachea to be breached and for oesophageal perforation to occur but careful technique during insertion should prevent this complication.

**Tracheostomy**. Tracheostomy is indicated when endotracheal intubation is impossible and long-term control of the airway is required. Tracheostomy tubes have a larger internal diameter than cricothyroidotomy tubes and their resistance to respiration is less. Use of a cuffed tracheostomy tube also protects the lower airway from soiling with blood or stomach contents. Unless all other methods fail, a tracheostomy is not indicated in the emergency situation because of the time it takes to gain control of the airway. Even in an emergency, some dissection is required before the trachea can be located and intubated.

# Additional factors affecting the management of upper airway obstruction

Gaining control of the airway in an injured patient is nearly always complicated by one or more problems. Simple solutions, logically applied, can reduce the need for the more complicated methods.

**Normal anatomical variants**. When preparing to administer general anaesthesia, anaesthetists automatically include in their preoperative assessment a search for anatomical features such as a receding chin, short thick neck or isolated canine teeth, which are known to be associated with difficult intubation. In the heat of an emergency, the more obvious airway problems caused by injury tend to gain most attention and anatomical variants are less likely to be noticed. In the injured patient these variants can turn a difficult intubation into an impossible one. Assessment of the airway in the injured patient should, therefore, include normal anatomical variants.

**The risk of vomiting and regurgitation**. The normal stomach takes between four and six hours to empty completely. As a normal meal is consumed, the stomach secretes acid and digestive juices. One hour after a meal, the volume of the stomach contents has doubled. Thereafter, the stomach empties and the volume of its contents decreases in an exponential fashion. Injury, alcohol, pain, opiate analgesics, fear and benzodiazepines reduce the rate of stomach emptying and, in combination, may stop emptying completely for 24 hours or more. In the injured patient, it is wise to assume that the stomach stopped emptying at the time of injury. The timing of the intake of food and drink in relation to the time of the injury gives the best guide to the likely volume of retained stomach contents. It is an unfortunate fact of life that most accidents occur within three hours of food and, in young adults, alcohol consumption. Perhaps because of this short time scale, the stomach contents of injured patients are often not as acidic as might be expected. The pulmonary inhalation of liquid stomach contents rarely causes significant pulmonary damage. The inhalation of solid stomach contents is more important because the lower airways may become blocked causing pulmonary collapse. If solid food is inhaled, bronchoscopy may be indicated. When anaesthesia is planned, precautions to reduce the risk of pulmonary aspiration can be taken (p. 104). In an emergency, cricoid pressure pressure is helpful but there is rarely time to empty the stomach, reduce the acidity of its contents or to inhibit the secretion of acid.

**Nasopharyngeal haemorrhage**. Patients with fractures to the base of the skull or the nose may bleed torrentially into the oropharynx. Continuous suction may be insufficient to keep the oropharynx clear. On indirect laryngoscopy, the larynx may be obscured by blood. If the larynx is visible, the view may subsequently be lost if blood covers the laryngoscope bulb. It may be possible to gain an accurate impression of the position of the larynx with one laryngoscope. Replacement of this laryngoscope with a clean one and positioning of the endotracheal tube in rapid sequence may solve the problem. If the bleeding is from fractured nasal bones and shows no sign of stopping spontaneously, a Foley catheter can be passed through each nostril. Having inflated the balloons with a small volume of air, tying the catheters together in front of the columella so that the balloons tamponade the posterior nasal space will often divert the flow of blood away from the oropharynx and hence improve the view on indirect laryngoscopy. If the bleeding is secondary to a basal skull fracture, the catheters should be passed with extreme caution as there is a risk that they will pass into the cranial cavity. This risk must be balanced against the risks of hypoxia and continued pulmonary inhalation of blood consequent on failure to achieve endotracheal intubation.

**Massive pulmonary oedema or haemorrhage**. Massive pulmonary oedema or haemorrhage may well up from the trachea into the oropharynx and obscure the view of the larynx. Sometimes the only clue to the location of the larynx is the presence of bubbles on expiration. A gum elastic bougie aimed at the bubbles may pass into the trachea. Alternatively, retrograde cannulation of the trachea and larynx with a long central venous catheter passed through the cricothyroid membrane can be helpful. The cannula is easily located in the mouth by touch or direct vision and an endotracheal tube can be threaded over it.

**The clenched jaw**. The clenched jaw may make the insertion of an oral airway or oral endotracheal tube extremely difficult. Use of the nasal route circumvents the problem of gaining access to the oral cavity. The clenched jaw is, however, often associated with the presence of obtunded but significant reflex activity of the airway. It may not be possible to pass a tube into the trachea without provoking, retching, vomiting or coughing. Vomiting is undesirable in any patient with obtunded reflexes, and particularly in this situation, when suctioning may also be difficult. Retching, vomiting and coughing are also undesirable in the patient with raised intracranial pressure. It is sometimes preferable to administer a general anaesthetic prior to endotracheal intubation. Provided that the anaesthetist does not render the patient apnoeic unless he is sure that the trachea can be intubated, the use of general anaesthesia often makes an uncontrolled and potentially tricky situation, easier. The risks of vomiting and pulmonary inhalation of gastric contents after general anaesthesia are probably less in this situation, than in the unanaesthetized patient.

**Cervical spine injury.** Quite rightly, all doctors faced with intubating a severely injured, unconscious patient, worry that an unstable cervical spine fracture may be present particularly if there are obvious injuries above the clavicle. If the spinal cord is damaged during intubation, the doctor has committed the patient to a life of quadriplegia and possibly ventilation. In the United Kingdom, the incidence of cervical spine injury is low. The incidence in patients with major trauma has not been well studied but is probably about one in a hundred patients. Not every patient with a cervical spine injury requires intubation. Even in busy trauma units, it is unlikely that a trainee anaesthetist will treat such a patient more than once or twice a year. This puts the problem in perspective. Every attempt should be made to immobilize the cervical spine until a fracture can be excluded radiographically. Several methods of immobilizing the cervical spine have already been described (p. 23). If a rigid collar is used mouth opening may be restricted. The collar should be removed and other methods of immobilization employed during intubation.

Ideally, all patients with a possible cervical spine injury should have cervical spine X-rays taken prior to intubation, but in the real world this is not always possible. The choice between nasal and oral endotracheal intubation has already been described (pp. 27–28). The crucial point is that the neck should not be moved from the neutral position. The choice of intubation method depends not only on the inherent advantages and disadvantages of the methods, but also on the skill and expertise of the anaesthetist. Both intubation methods should be practised on resuscitation dummies and in the controlled environment of the anaesthetic room. The anaesthetist should then be able to make a reasoned decision about the best technique to employ in the A&E department. When intubating a severely injured patient, the anaesthetist would do well to remember that cervical spine injury is relatively rare but unconsciousness due to head injury is common. This thought may give some comfort but should not allow complacency. While every attempt should be made to avoid damage to the spinal cord, simultaneous efforts must be made to ensure that the patient does not become hypoxic during intubation. The outcome after head injury is worsened by any hypoxic episode.

**Maxillofacial injuries**.  Maxillofacial injuries are often impressive in appearance but rarely cause significant airway problems in the immediate post-injury period. The anatomy of the oropharynx is usually preserved. Fractures to the mandible and maxilla often improve mouth opening which only becomes restricted when oedema and muscle spasm develop several hours after injury. The biggest problem is haemorrhage. Prior to admisssion to hospital, the conscious patient will usually have adopted a position which permits drainage of blood to the exterior. If there is loss of airway control and protection due to a concomitant head injury, bleeding can be a significant problem. In this situation, intubation of the trachea is mandatory. If intubation is impossible, a tracheostomy is essential. A tracheostomy is often required after definitive maxillofacial surgery but this should not deter the anaesthetist from attempting endotracheal intubation in the emergency situation.

# The causes and diagnosis of respiratory insufficiency

Abnormal breathing, better described as respiratory insufficiency has five pathophysiological causes. These are summarized in Table 1.2.1. During resuscitation, treatment of the deranged physiology is life saving. An accurate clinical diagnosis can be delayed until the secondary survey is complete.

**UPPER AIRWAY OBSTRUCTION** (Table 1.1.1, p. 13 and pp. 20–21)

**Inadequate or inappropriate movement of the chest wall**. The most common cause for inadequate movement of the chest wall is pain. Frequently this is due to rib fractures but it may also be due to sternal fractures, severe bruising or an open, sucking wound. Sometimes patients with abdominal injuries breathe shallowly as this reduces their abdominal pain. Abdominal distention and diaphragmatic injury restrict diaphragmatic movement.

Chest wall movement may be reduced in an asymmetrical fashion if the underlying lung is collapsed secondary to a pneumothorax or plug in a major airway. If individual ribs are fractured in two places, a flail segment is seen which moves paradoxically to the rest of the chest wall. If a pneumothorax is present, the percussion note is hyper-resonant. In the case of pulmonary collapse due to a plug, the percussion note is dull. This should not be confused with the dull percussion note heard over a haemothorax. The two can be distinguished by rolling the patient. Unless the haemothorax is massive, in which case there will also be signs of hypovolaemia, the area of dullness moves to the dependent area of the pleural cavity. In most cases of respiratory insufficiency, there is time to take a chest X-ray to confirm the diagnosis. The exception to this rule is the presence of a tension pneumothorax in which one lung totally collapses causing severe hypoxia. Distortion of the mediastinum may simultaneously cause occlusion of the vena cavae, reduced venous return, engorgement of the jugular veins, suffusion of the face and neck, and cardiovascular collapse.

**Table 1.2.1 Causes of respiratory insufficiency and hypoxia following injury**

1. Upper airway obstruction (Table 1.1.1, p. 13)

2. Inadequate or inappropriate chest wall excursion
   (a) simple rib fractures
   (b) flail segment
   (c) soft tissue injury
   (d) sternal fracture
   (e) diaphragmatic rupture
   (f) spinal cord transection
   (g) open sucking chest wound
   (h) diaphragmatic splinting

3. Inadequate lung expansion
   (a) inadequate chest wall excursion
   (b) pneumothorax
   (c) haemothorax
   (d) injury to trachea or bronchus
   (e) foreign body in a major airway
   (f) pulmonary contusion
   (h) abdominal contents

4. Abnormal respiratory drive
   (a) head injury
   (b) severe hypoxia
   (c) severe hypovolaemia
   (d) metabolic acidosis secondary to hypoxia
   (e) alcohol or drug intoxication

5. Impaired gas exchange
   (a) pulmonary contusion
   (b) pulmonary aspiration of blood or stomach contents
   (c) pulmonary collapse secondary to pneumothorax, haemothorax, sputum plug or foreign body
   (d) pulmonary oedema
   (e) inadequate perfusion due to hypovolaemia, myocardial failure, microemboli or microthrombi

**Inadequate lung expansion.** Lung expansion is reduced by inadequate movement of the chest wall. It may also be restricted by air or blood in the pleural cavity. During spontaneous respiration, abdominal contents may be sucked into the pleural cavity through a diaphragmatic rupture. Upper or lower airway obstruction also reduces gas flow to the lungs. Lower airway obstruction is less common than upper airway obstruction but can just as easily cause hypoxia. It may be due to inhalation of blood clot, solid food or foreign bodies. Rarely, bronchial or tracheal tears cause reduced airflow to the lungs. The correct diagnosis should be made by observing chest wall movement, percussion and auscultation of the lungs. Radiological examination may provide confirmation of the diagnosis.

**Abnormal respiratory drive**.    The brain stem is responsible for the central control of respiration. Direct injury to the brain stem is rare but the respiratory pattern can be disturbed by cerebral swelling, primary hypoxia or hypoxia secondary to hypovolaemia. Chronic bronchitics may be dependent on hypoxia for their respiratory drive. Cerebral depression is also caused by alcoholic intoxication.

There are also peripheral stimulae which have an effect on respiratory drive. In particular, the arterial pH is important. A significant acidosis may increase the respiratory rate to inefficiently high levels.

**Impaired gas exchange**.    The transfer of gas across the alveolar capillary membrane may be reduced by blood and secretions in the alveoli which obscure the alveolar membrane or by disruption of the alveolar–capillary membrane as a result of primary injury or the inhalation of acidic stomach contents. The diagnosis should be suspected if there is a history of chest injury or inhalation of blood or stomach contents. The diagnosis can be confirmed if secretions, stomach contents or blood are aspirated from the trachea during suction. There may also be opacities on the chest X-ray but the absence of radiological changes in the first hour after injury does not necessarily exclude the diagnosis. Pulmonary contusion or interstitial oedema secondary to acid damage may not be apparent radiologically for up to eight hours after injury.

Inadequate pulmonary blood flow reduces the amount of oxygen carrying haemoglobin in the capillaries so that, even if transfer across the alveolar capillary membrane is adequate, there may be insufficient blood to carry oxygen to the tissues. Blood flow in the capillaries may be reduced by absolute hypovolaemia due to haemorrhage or relative hypovolaemia caused by spinal injury, cardiac tamponade or a tension pneumothorax. Flow may also be reduced by microemboli from bone marrow fat or the debris in stored blood products.

Further reductions in blood flow to the lungs can be caused by over-zealous mechanical ventilation. Excessive mean intrathoracic pressures will reduce venous return and hence pulmonary blood flow.

In the presence of inadequate pulmonary blood flow, severe tissue hypoxia will occur, no matter how well the lungs are ventilated. The diagnosis should be suspected in the presence of any injuries which cause bleeding and hypovolaemia (Table 1.2.2, p. 43). Microemboli may also reduce pulmonary blood flow but their presence can only be confirmed at post mortem. If the patient is being mechanically ventilated, the ventilator settings should be checked and particular attention paid to the inflation pressure and mean intrathoracic pressure.

# General principles for the management of respiratory insufficiency

The management of respiratory insufficiency depends on the recognition of the pathophysiological changes which are present. The administration of pure oxygen is beneficial while the diagnosis is being made and other treatment being administered. If the patient's condition allows it, simple measures should be attempted first.

**Analgesia**.   Pain relief should always be administered as soon as is reasonably possible. Some suitable methods are discussed on pp. 76–80.

**Restoration of circulating blood volume**.   This topic is discussed on pp. 67–68 and 70–71.

**Drainage of the pleural cavity**.   Sucking wounds should be sealed with an occlusive dressing. Drainage of air from the pleural cavity will permit full expansion of the lungs. There are some who believe that it is preferable to allow small pneumothoraces to re-absorb naturally. In a few uncomplicated cases, this is probably an acceptable approach. Before deciding not to insert a chest drain, it is wise to take into consideration other factors such as the potential need for mechanical ventilation or a general anaestheic using nitrous oxide and the presence of a head injury in which even a minor degree of hypoxia may worsen the eventual outcome. If the pneumothorax is small and the leak seals quickly, it is often possible to remove chest drains within 24 hours of insertion. If there is any doubt, it is preferable to drain air from the pleural cavity.

The presence of a visible haemothorax on the chest X-ray usually means that the pleural cavity contains at least one litre of blood. Not only does this blood impede lung expansion, but also it may form a solid haematoma which has the potential to become infected. Visible haemothoraces should be drained. Continuing blood loss can be monitored after drainage of the original haemothorax and if the loss is less than 200 ml in a 24-hour period, the chest drain can be removed. Hourly losses from a chest drain of 400 ml or more for several hours may be an indication for thoracotomy.

**Controlled mechanical ventilation**.   If there is any doubt about the adequacy of ventilation, or if the measures described above are insufficient to relieve respiratory insufficiency, mechanical ventilation is mandatory. Initially 100 % oyxgen should be given and the tidal and minute volumes should be chosen so that, with each inspiratory breath, there is visible but not excessive excursion of the chest wall. When life-saving measures have been completed and definitive management is being planned, the ventilatory pattern and inspired oxygen concentration can be determined by the nature of the injuries and the adequacy of arterial oxygenation.

**Double lumen tubes**.   There is little, if any, place for the use of a double lumen tube in the relief of respiratory insufficiency during life-saving resuscitation. The only possible exception might be if there is a penetrating chest injury which is undubitably unilateral and has caused a significant bronchopulmonary injury. The respiratory distress in this type of injury is due either to a massive air leak or to torrential intrapulmonary haemorrhage. Isolation of the injured lung, and ventilation of the uninjured lung, may be the only method of ensuring oxygenation although hypoxia is unlikely to be relieved completely. In practise, it is rarely possible to be certain of the path of a penetrating wound or the precise extent of any pulmonary injury. If the patient is ill enough to require immediate intubation, it is preferable to ventilate through a standard single lumen endotracheal tube. If this proves insufficient, bronchoscopy will clarify the diagnosis. If the patient is in extremis, an emergency room thoracotomy is often the only option.

# Difficulties in the management of respiratory insufficiency

**The decision to commence ventilation**.   Ventilation should be commenced if the patient is obviously cyanosed, if respiratory effort is minimal or obviously grossly abnormal and if the patient is apnoeic. The causes of respiratory insufficiency are numerous and have been discussed previously. If there is any doubt about the adequacy of respiration, the patient should be intubated and ventilated immediately. There are, however, dangers associated with intubation and ventilation. The complications of mechanical ventilation include barotrauma, sepsis, accidental disconnection, ventilator failure and reduced venous return. For these reasons, mechanical ventilation should not be undertaken lightly. It is possible to gently manually ventilate a patient through a face mask. Gastric distention and regurgitation of stomach contents may occur. Some protection to the airway can be provided by the application of cricoid pressure. Manual ventilation should normally only be considered if the period of ventilation required is likely to be extremely brief. This situation is rare but might occur in a grossly hypovolaemic patient who has bled from peripheral injuries. The method is mandatory if the patient is in need of ventilation and cannot be intubated immediately.

In less urgent situations, the criterion for ventilation should be a progressive deterioration in the patient's condition which is not responding to other forms of treatment. Methods of monitoring the adequacy of oxygenation and ventilation are described on pp. 57, 61 and 63. The anaesthetist should utilize all the information available to him. Traditionally, formal measurements are made at 5-, 10- or 15-minute intervals during the resuscitation period. The anaesthetist should, however, be continually aware of the patient's appearance. Subtle deteriorations may be apparent to the skilled clinician but may not be measurable by monitoring devices. Equally, a dramatic deterioration may develop in seconds rather than minutes.

**Inability to ventilate the lungs**.   Fortunately, this is a rare problem in the seriously injured patient. More commonly, the lungs can be ventilated but excessive pressures are required. All the usual causes of difficulty with ventilation which are encountered in the anaesthetized patient should be considered. If the patient can be ventilated manually, the problem lies with the ventilator. If the patient cannot be ventilated manually, the circuit and endotracheal tube should be checked for obstruction. The problem is most likely to be with the endotracheal tube which may be blocked by a herniated cuff. If deflation of the cuff does not cure the problem, a sucker should be passed down the tube. If it does not pass freely, the tube is blocked. The obstruction may be due to kinking or to a blood clot in the tube. The tube should be changed. It may be possible to pass a gum elastic bougie down the tube, even though a sucker will not pass. If this can be done and a new tube railroaded over the bougie, this is helpful, particularly if the initial intubation was difficult. If the problem is still present, the cause lies distal to the tube. It could be due to severe bronchospasm in an asthmatic patient or aspiration of acid stomach contents.

In the severely injured patient, inability to ventilate the lungs may be due to an intrathoracic tracheal or bronchial rupture, both of which are associated with massive air leaks. A double lumen tube may solve the problem. It may also be due to the presence of large blood clots in the trachea or main stem bronchi or to the inhalation of food or a foreign body prior to admission to hospital. Bronchoscopic removal may be indicated. If there is distortion of the trachea due to a tension pneumothorax or mediastinal haematoma, the tip of the endotracheal tube may impinge on the tracheal wall. Rotation of the tube or withdrawal by a few centimetres may help until definitive treatment is given. If it is totally impossible to ventilate the lungs and the problem is known to be distal to the endotracheal tube and amenable to surgical treatment, this is an indication for emergency room thoracotomy. Alternatively, if the trachea has been damaged by a penetrating injury to the neck and the trachea is visible through the wound, intubation and ventilation can be effected through the wound.

**Inability to achieve adequate arterial oxygenation**. This situation is grave if it is encountered during the resuscitation period and cannot be corrected. The oxygen delivery system should be checked to ensure that 100% oxygen is being correctly administered. The adequacy of ventilation should also be checked and, if possible, cardiovascular parameters normalized. If these measures fail, positive end expiratory pressure should be tried bearing in mind the increased risk of barotrauma and the fact that the rise in intrathoracic pressure may cause a secondary rise in intracranial pressure or a decrease in venous return.

Patients who remain severely hypoxic, in spite of adequate resuscitation and definitive treatment, generally have a poor outcome. The exception to this rule is when hypoxia is due to the inhalation of a large amount of blood.

# The causes and diagnosis of cardiovascular insufficiency

There are six major causes of cardiovascular collapse after injury. These are summarized in Table 1.2.2. Failure to recognize and treat the cause of cardiovascular collapse will usually have fatal consequences. Life-threatening cardiovascular collapse may be recognized by the absence of at least two major pulses. Major pulses may be palpated over the carotid, axillary or femoral arteries. It is preferable to palpate the pulse at two sites because the absence of a pulse at a single site may be due to local injury or circulatory pathology.

**Major haemorrhage**.   Cardiovascular collapse due to acute blood loss is likely to occur if the blood volume is reduced by more than 40%. In the average 70 kg male, a 40% reduction

**Table 1.2.2 Causes of cardiovascular collapse following injury**

1.  Cardiac arrest
2.  Major haemorrhage
3.  Cardiac tamponade
4.  Tension pneumothorax
5.  Massive head injury
6.  Myocardial failure due to contusion, infarction or dysrhythmias

in blood volume is equivalent to a loss of at least two litres of blood. There are individual patient variations. Notably, the old and infirm are less able to tolerate blood loss and athletes are capabable of tolerating greater losses than normal individuals. The rapidity of blood loss and time since injury also affect the response. In response to hypovolaemia, the patient appears pale, the pulse rate and respiratory rate rise, the blood pressure and pulse pressure fall, vasoconstriction causes reduced capillary filling, collapsed veins, confusion or loss of consciousness, and minimal or absent urine output. Lesser volumes of blood loss produce similar but less dramatic changes in the parameters of cardiovascular status. These are summarized in Table 1.2.3.

Almost any injury can be associated with significant blood loss (pp. 67–68). Although some injuries cause relatively insignificant blood loss, a combination of two or more of these injuries may cause losses normally associated with more major injuries.

**Cardiac arrest**. Cardiac arrest is the second commonest cause of cardiovascular collapse in the injured patient. It is usually due to exsanguination, untreated cardiac tamponade or tension pneumothorax, massive head injury, cervical spinal cord injury, or massive tracheobronchial disruption. Rarely, it is due to a myocardial infarction which precipitated the accident. In theory, cardiac arrest prior to admission to

**Table 1.2.3 Physiological responses to acute blood loss in adults**

| Blood loss | <1500 ml | 1500–2000 ml | >2000 ml |
|---|---|---|---|
| Heart rate (bpm) | 80–120 | 120–140 | >140 |
| Systolic BP (mmHg) | 120 | 70–90 | <70 |
| Peripheral vasoconstriction | + −++ | +++ | +++ |
| Urine output (ml/h) | >50 | 20–50 | 0–20 |
| Mental status | Mild anxiety | Anxious or confused | Confused or reduced conscious level |

hospital could be due to hypoxia secondary to untreated airway obstruction, but training of the general public and emergency personnel in emergency care has virtually banished this cause to the history books. A scheme for diagnosing the cause of cardiac arrest is shown in Table 1.2.4.

**Cardiac tamponade**. Cardiac tamponade normally occurs after a deceleration injury or penetrating chest injury. Typically the patient appears well until the blood pressure suddenly falls. The heart rate increases and the neck veins become engorged. The upper trunk, neck and face appear suffused and purple. Heart sounds become muffled. The lungs sound normal on percussion and auscultation which should exclude the alternative diagnosis of tension pneumothorax. Classically, the heart appears globular on a chest X-ray, but if the patient is collapsed it is inappropriate to delay treatment for radiological confirmation of the diagnosis.

There are two events which, although not diagnostic of cardiac tamponade or scientifically validated, should alert the clinician to the possibility of impending tamponade, particularly if the type of accident is known to be compatible with this injury. Both occur when the patient is apparently well and is not thought to have a serious injury. Firstly, the patient may become subjectively short of breath and will struggle to sit up. There are no clinical findings to explain why the patient complains of breathlessness. Secondly, the patient may have a premonition of impending disaster and informs the doctors that he is sure he is going to die. Again, the clinical signs do not confirm this fear. In the author's experience, these subjective events are commonly followed, within a few minutes, by cardiovascular collapse due to cardiac tamponade.

**Tension pneumothorax**. Some of the clinical signs of tension pneumothorax are similar to those of cardiac tamponade; the blood pressure falls and the neck veins become distended. The differential diagnosis is not hard to make provided that other clinical signs of a tension pneumothorax

**Table 1.2.4 The diagnosis and management of cardiovascular collapse in injured patients**

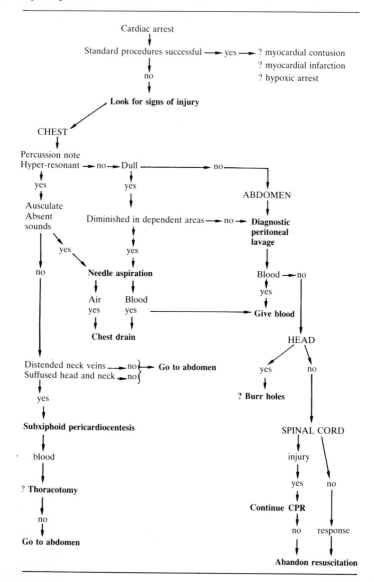

are sought. The trachea is deviated away from the side of the pneumothorax, the percussion note is hyper-resonant and the breath sounds are absent on the side of the pneumo-thorax. There is usually a history of a direct blow to the ribs and rib fractures may be diagnosed clinically, even though they are not apparent radiologically. The X-ray findings are classical showing air in the pleural cavity, a collapsed lung, deviation of the trachea and shift of the mediastinal contents away from the side of the pneumothorax. As with cardiac tamponade, treatment should not be delayed while radiolo-gical confirmation of the diagnosis is awaited.

**Myocardial failure**. Myocardial contusion can occur with any chest injury but is most common in vehicle drivers who are thrown against the steering wheel. It is very rare for myocardial contusion to be severe enough to be the sole cause of cardiovascular collapse. Clinical signs are usually minimal. There may be a steering wheel imprint on the chest wall or other marks indicating injury to the anterior chest wall. The electrocardiogram may show ST segment elevation or dysrhythmias. The diagnosis cannot be confirmed or denied during the resuscitation period.

Sometimes accidents occur due to the acute onset of a medical illness. Of these illnesses, myocardial infarction is most likely to cause cardiovascular collapse. The clinical findings are limited to ECG changes similar to those seen in myocardial contusion. A history of heart disease or a bottle of glyceryl trinitrate tablets found amongst the patient's belongings may provide clues to the diagnosis.

**Massive head injury**. Severe head injury causing direct damage to the brain stem or cerebral oedema sufficient to cause coning will disrupt the function of the cardiovascular control centre. Usually, this is manifest as wild swings in pulse rate and blood pressure associated with a variety of dysrhythmias. Very rarely, the injury is severe enough to cause bradycardia and hypotension which are followed rapidly by cardiac arrest.

Hypotension accompanied by tachycardia in the head injured patient should *never* be assumed to be due to the head injury. It is usually due to hypovolaemia secondary to haemorrhage. If the hypovolaemia is not treated, a favourable outcome from the head injury is impossible.

# General management principles for cardiovascular insufficiency

The management of cardiovascular collapse depends on the diagnosis and is summarized in Table 1.2.4 (p. 46). In every case, it is vital to secure venous access as rapidly as possible. Because major haemorrhage is the most likely cause of the collapse, large bore cannulae should be placed above and below the diaphragm. This means that blood can be infused via the superior and inferior vena cava. Bleeding in the region of drainage of either part of the cava can then be replaced.

**Hypovolaemia.** All patients should be given oxygen. Visible sources of bleeding should be controlled. Usually, a pressure dressing is sufficient. Occasionally, direct digital pressure over the bleeding site is necessary. Pressure on the femoral or axillary arteries will often control bleeding in the relevant limb. A tourniquet or arterial clamp should be used as a last resort to control haemorrhage as the potential for additional damage to the blood vessels by the equipment is often greater than is justified by the severity of bleeding.

It is vital that the circulating blood volume is restored as quickly as possible. While blood is being crossmatched, a standard regime should be used. The precise regime is less important than the speed with which it is administered. Many centres have a protocol governing fluid management. In the United Kingdom, the protocol usually suggests that 1 or 2 litres of physiological saline solution be administered, followed by $1\frac{1}{2}$ litres of an isotonic colloid solution such as human albumin solution, Haemaccel® or Gelofusin®. If the rapid infusion of these fluids does not restore the systolic blood pressure to at least 90 mmHg, group O-negative blood is transfused until type-specific or saline crossmatched blood is available. All fluids should be warmed. Most seriously injured patients are already hypothermic by the time they are admitted to hospital. Removal of clothes for assessment of the injuries and treatment usually results in further heat loss. There is evidence to suggest that hypothermia, independent of the type of injuries, increases the ultimate mortality rate.

For patients with continuing haemorrhage from a pelvic fracture or intra-abdominal injury and in whom it is impossible to transfuse blood at a sufficient ratè to maintain blood pressure, the application of a pneumatic antishock garment can be helpful. These garments take time to apply and must not be used at the expense of continuing transfusion of fluid. Their use is contraindicated if there is bleeding outside the confines of the garment, the patient has a ruptured diaphragm or has pulmonary oedema, with or without left ventricular dysfunction.

**Cardiac tamponade**.   Blood should be aspirated from the pericardial sac using a long needle inserted 2 cm below the left xiphichondral junction and inserted at a 45° angle to the skin aiming towards the tip of the left scapula. If the patient is conscious, local anaesthetic may be required for the skin and subcutaneous tissues. Usually, aspiration of 20 or 30 ml of blood will be sufficient to raise the blood pressure and temporarily stabilize the patient's condition for long enough to permit transfer to the operating theatre for a formal thoracotomy. An emergency room thoracotomy is rarely, if ever, indicated for cardiac tamponade.

**Tension pneumothorax**.   As an emergency measure, a plastic intravenous cannula can be inserted into the pleural cavity. Air will be heard to hiss out of the cannula as the tension is released. Not only will the life-threatening nature of the problem be temporarily removed, but also the diagnosis will be confirmed. When the situation has been temporarily controlled in this way, the needle can be removed after a chest drain connected to an underwater seal has been inserted under sterile conditions using local anaesthesia.

**Myocardial failure**.   As a temporary life-saving measure, inotropic agents may be given. Initially, dobutamine is probably the drug of choice but dopamine or noradrenaline may also be useful. In an emergency, treatment will be guided by the reponse of the pulse and blood pressure. As soon as the patient's life is no longer in danger, a pulmonary artery flotation catheter should be inserted. This will give information about filling pressures, cardiac output and oxygen flux and is a far more accurate and effective method of monitoring treatment than a central venous pressure catheter.

If heart failure is due to dysrhythmias, management should be directed towards their control. Sometimes, myocardial contusion or an infarct damage the ventricular septum and cause complete heart block. Cardiac pacing is indicated. In the acute situation, rapid control of atrial fibrillation or flutter can be achieved by cardioversion. Drug therapy is usually reserved for repeated episodes of a dysrhythmia (pp. 192–194).

The management of myocardial failure is discussed in greater detail on pp. 199–201. In a medical emergency, there may be a little time to consider various treatment options. For the seriously injured patient, delays in treatment are critical because there may be other factors which also threaten tissue oxygenation. Treatment is therefore selected because it will produce the most rapid results and because it will have the least impact on the management of other injuries.

**Massive head injury**.   The treatment of serious head injuries is discussed on pp. 86–91. It is extremely unusual for treatment to have any impact on the blood pressure if the cardiovascular collapse is genuinely due to the head injury. Consideration should be given to the use of inotropes. The improvement in blood pressure does not reflect an improvement in prognosis, which is usually hopeless. Maintenance of organ perfusion does, however, delay death and allow the relatives time to consider the possibility of organ donation. If there are multiple injuries and organ donation is not an option, there is no point in prolonging the process of dying by administering inotropes.

**Cardiac arrest.** Initially, the management of cardiac arrest in the injured patient is no different to the management of cardiac arrest in other patients (pp. 182–185). Restoration of effective cardiac rhythm is, however, unlikely to be successful unless the cause of the arrest is also diagnosed and treated concurrently with the normal cardiac arrest procedures.

# *Difficulties in the management of cardiovascular insufficiency*

In the severely injured patient, there are three primary difficulties in the management of cardiovascular collapse. The first, and most common, is inability to secure rapid venous access. In the absence of venous access, it is impossible to initiate treatment. The second problem is the inability to secure an improvement in the patient's clinical condition despite appropriate treatment. The third, which has implications for the second, is the inability to make the correct diagnosis.

**Inability to secure venous access.** Securing venous access should never be a real problem provided that the anaesthetist has anticipated the likely problems and has mastered various techniques in the controlled situation of the anaesthetic room and the intensive care unit. Intense vasoconstriction occurs in response to major haemorrhage. Peripheral veins are frequently collapsed. In addition, vasoconstricion occurs in response to cold, pain and anxiety, all of which are common in injured patients. Furthermore, access to peripheral veins may be limited by lacerations, grazes and fractures. In the severely injured patient, it is vital to secure venous access rapidly. Ideally, the site of access should be away from joints and into a large peripheral vein. This can be difficult to achieve because of the problems already mentioned. In experienced hands, cannulation of the central veins is just as quick as peripheral venous cannulation and is not hampered by vasoconstriction. Before treating seriously injured patients, all doctors should make themselves competent in cannulating two central veins. One of these veins should be above and the other below the diaphragm. Below the diaphragm, there is only one choice. The femoral vein is constant in position and lies 1 cm medial to the femoral artery. Unless the patient is moribund, it is usually possible to palpate the pulse of the femoral artery with reasonable ease. If the pulse is impalpable, its anatomical location is reasonably constant, being midway along a line drawn between the symphysis pubis and the anterior iliac spines. In routine anaesthetic practice, cannulation of the femoral vessels is frowned upon because of the proximity of the perineum and anus and the potential risks of infection. The anaesthetist is, therefore, advised to practise this technique on carefully selected patients. It is a remarkably easy technique to learn, and most anaesthetists should require only one or two practice cannulations to gain confidence for the emergency situation.

Above the diaphragm, there is a greater choice of sites. For uninjured patients, cannulation of the internal jugular vein is often preferred because there is said to be less risk of pleural puncture than when the subclavian vein is used. For the resuscitation of the seriously injured patient, cannulation of the subclavian vein has much to commend it. The most important reason for choosing this site is that movement of the neck is not necessary. As with endotracheal intubation, the risks of moving the neck must always be considered prior to internal jugular vein cannulation. All central venous sites above the diaphragm have clear anatomical landmarks to aid cannulation so that cardiovascular collapse or cardiac arrest should not delay the establishment of venous access.

Non-anaesthetists are often taught that if peripheral venous cannulation fails, the next option is venous cut down in the groin, ankle or antecubital fossa. All anaesthetists should be familiar with this technique but, even in skilled hands, it takes time to establish venous access in this manner. It should probably be reserved for patients in whom other methods are impossible or have failed.

In the severely hypovolaemic patient, it is vital that blood can be given rapidly in order to replace pre-existing losses and to keep up with continuing losses. Flow through a tube is reduced in proportion to increasing length and increased in proportion to the fourth power of an increase in radius. When choosing a cannula, consideration should be given not only to its bore but also to its length. The introducer kits intended for pulmonary artery flotation catheters are ideal for rapid transfusion of blood because they are relatively short and have a wide bore. In some centres, the end of an intravenous giving set is cut off and the giving set is inserted into the femoral vein under direct vision in the erroneous belief that this will permit even greater rates of transfusion. The rate of flow for a giving set is, however, dependent on and limited by the size of the orifice into the drip chamber. In many giving sets, this is little different from the size of a pulmonary artery flotation catheter introducer.

**Failure to gain a satisfactory response to treatment**.   There are three causes for this problem. Firstly, if the patient is hypovolaemic, blood administration may be too slow. This may be because the cannulae are too small or there are not enough of them. Secondly, bleeding may be so rapid that it is impossible to keep up with losses even when several large bore cannulae are used. In this situation, surgical control of bleeding is mandatory. Once the bleeding vessel has been clamped, definitive treatment can proceed simultaneously with resuscitation. In the case of profuse haemorrhage from a pelvic fracture or intra-abdominal injury, the pneumatic anti-shock garment can, with the provisos mentioned on

p. 49, be used to gain temporary respite. Thirdly, all injuries may not have been diagnosed and hence the volume of the blood transfusion is insufficient and inappropriate. Soft tissue injuries, for example, can cause massive blood loss but if this is distributed along tissue planes, may not cause obvious swelling.

**Failure to make the correct diagnosis**.   Sometimes the response to an apparently adequate transfusion is disappointing. The usual explanation is that the patient's injuries have been incompletely or inadequately diagnosed. If the clinical signs suggest continuing hypovolaemia, occult bleeding into the abdomen or chest should be suspected. Clinical examination of the chest for progressive dullness to percussion and a chest X-ray should identify occult bleeding. The abdomen may be visibly distending but significant bleeding does not always cause abdominal distension. A diagnostic peritoneal lavage or ultrasound examination of the abdomen is helpful at this stage.

If continuing hypotension is not due to inadequately treated haemorrhage, consideration should be given to the possible coexistence of other causes of cardiovascular collapse such as cardiac tamponade, tension pneumothorax or severe head injury. It is also possible that age, physical fitness or medication such as beta blockers or calcium antagonists may be causing an atypical response to haemorrhage.

# *Monitoring life-saving resuscitation*

The monitoring methods chosen for the resuscitation period are not normally as sophisticated as those used during complex anaesthesia or intensive care. There are two possible scenarios when a seriously injured patient is admitted to the A&E department. The first is that a doctor is assessing and treating the patient single handed. In this case, there is no time to insert lines for invasive monitoring. In fact, most monitoring will be initiated by the nursing staff. The second scenario is that a team of doctors is assessing and treating the patient. In this case there is rarely room for more than three doctors to work on the patient at one time. The first will be securing the airway and establishing satisfactory ventilation, the second will be establishing intravenous access and starting fluid replacement and the third will be examining the patient. Monitoring techniques must be easy and quick to employ and, therefore, will be non-invasive. As resuscitation progresses, there may be an opportunity to proceed to invasive arterial and central venous pressure monitoring. The anaesthetist will, however, still be competing with medical colleagues who are performing a more detailed clinical examination, inserting urinary and possibly peritoneal lavage catheters and with radiographers who are taking the initial set of diagnostic X-rays. The anaesthetist will, in all probability, have to rely on basic monitoring techniques until the initial resuscitation period is over. As sophisticated, electronic, invasive monitoring devices have become available, there has been a tendency to abandon simple techniques in the erroneous belief that the information obtained is more valuable. If basic techniques are used to their full advantage by doctors with experience of their use, it is surprising how accurately initial resuscitation can be performed. As resuscitation progresses, additional monitoring methods can be employed to assist with the fine-tuning of fluid balance. Finally, when the patient has been stabilized, there may be a place for the use of a pulmonary artery flotation catheter but the measurements obtained should only be useful for the fine tuning of fluid balance and as a guide to the types and doses of inotropic drugs being used to support the myocardium.

The methods of monitoring available to the anaesthetist are described below. None of the techniques are infallible. All must be interpreted in the light of clinical findings and the information obtained from other monitoring techniques.

It follows that the more information that can be obtained, the more likely the interpretation is to be correct.

**Eyes, nose, ears and hands**.   Look at the patient. There may be signs of upper airway obstruction (pp. 20–21), abnormal or asymmetrical chest movement (p. 35), facial injuries, bleeding from the nose or ears, vomit on the patient or pillows, lack of response to stimulae or a penetrating wound to the neck or chest. All these might indicate airway or breathing difficulties. Look also for pallor, sweating, peripheral cyanosis, and overt haemorrhage which may suggest hypovolaemia. Conversely, distended neck veins may suggest adequate venous filling or, if grossly distended, the presence of cardiac tamponade or a tension pneumothorax.

Smell the patient. Alcohol on the breath may account for the patient's behaviour and will certainly delay stomach emptying. Alcohol is also an excellent analgesic agent which may mask pain from injury. Having made a provisional diagnosis of alcohol intoxication, the anaesthetist should always look for other injuries, particularly those causing an alteration in conscious level.

Listen for vocalization which gives clues to the level of consciousness and for grunting, gurgling from the throat or stridor which imply airway obstruction. Listen also to what the patient says about pain or to his cries as the clinical examination progresses. The presence of pain may give clues to the location of injuries, potential breathing difficulties and the possibility of significant haemorrhage.

Feel for warm air on expiration and the temperature of the limbs. This will give clues about the patency of the airway and adequacy of the peripheral circulation. Feel for the pulse to assess its rate, regularity and strength. This will give clues to the presence of hypovolaemia and dysrhythmias before the heart rate, blood pressure and electrocardiogram are monitored formally. Feel also for tenderness of the cervical spine or an abnormal spinal contour which may indicate a fracture. Palpate the trachea to assess its position and palpate the chest wall for surgical emphysema indicating an air leak or tenderness indicating rib fractures.

**Pulse oximetry**.   A pulse oximeter can easily be applied and measures the oxygen saturation at the site it is applied. Under normal circumstances, the reading obtained is very similar to that of arterial blood. The severely injured patient is not normal. Total erythrocyte volume and cardiac output may be reduced to a level where tissue hypoxia is a problem but the pulse oximeter may give no indication of these important problems if the remaining haemoglobin is well saturated. Peripheral vasoconstriction due to hypovolaemia, hypothermia, pain and anxiety will reduce the saturation of the peripheral circulation. Measurements of saturation may be low even though the patient is well oxygenated. Furthermore, because the upper part of the oxygen saturation curve is relatively flat, the oxygen saturation does not fall significantly until the arterial oxygen tension is severely reduced.

If, as has been recommended, oxygen is given to all severely injured patients from the time of admission, most patients will have oxygen saturations of 95% or more. If a sudden deterioration in the patient's condition occurs due to cardiac tamponade or a tension pneumothorax, it may take several minutes for the peripheral blood to become desaturated. Normal saturations, therefore, do not necessarily imply that all is well.

**Non-invasive pulse and blood pressure**.   Used in combination, measurements of the pulse rate and blood pressure can be very helpful. A normal pulse rate and blood pressure indicates that the vascular space is adequately filled, that the patient is pain free and that he is well oxygenated. It should not be forgotten, however, that these measures reflect the filling of the vascular space as it exists at the time of the measurement. In the normal healthy adult, intense vasoconstriction can compensate for losses of up to $1\frac{1}{2}$ litres of fluid. The patient is not in imminent danger, but may still be hypovolaemic. A rapid heart rate with reduced blood pressure normally indicates severe hypovolaemia but also occurs with cardiac tamponade, tension pneumothorax, myocardial failure or, rarely, severe pain. A progressively slowing pulse rate with increasing blood pressure indicates rising intracranial pressure. The process of brain stem death is accompanied by chaotic and frequent changes in pulse and blood pressure.

**Capillary and venous filling**. In the presence of vasoconstriction, capillary refill is slow. The veins are collapsed, which can make the placement of intravenous cannulae difficult. Hypovolaemia, hypothermia, pain and anxiety are common in severely injured patients. All cause an increase in sympathetic tone and slowed capillary refill. Severe head injury is also associated with increased activity of the sympathetic nervous system which causes peripheral vasoconstriction and, in its severest form, neurogenic pulmonary oedema. For this reason, normal capillary refill and distended peripheral veins should be regarded with suspicion in the patient with obvious, severe injuries. These signs could be one of the first clues suggesting spinal cord injury.

**Skin-core temperature difference**. The normal difference between the core temperature measured in the nasopharynx or oesophagus and the skin temperature of the great toe is less than 2°C. Anything which causes vasoconstriction will increase this difference. Furthermore, the peripheral temperature which is measured is solely that of the great toe. The great toe skin to core temperature difference is nearly always greater than normal and its use during resuscitation is virtually valueless. It is far better to feel the patient's skin. A cold great toe means very little. A cold foot indicates moderate vasoconstriction, whilst a cold limb up to the knee indicates severe vasoconstriction. In the absence of hypothermia and pain, cold skin up to the knee usually means that the blood volume is depleted by at least 2 litres.

**Urine output**. A decrease in urine output is always a significant finding because it usually occurs in the presence of hypovolaemia severe enough to cause vasoconstriction of the renal vascular bed. It can also occur as a result of primary injury to the renal tract. In this instance, blood is seen or detected biochemically in the urine. Rarely, a severe crush injury releases myoglobin from the muscles. The urine darkens and may be reduced in volume. Absent urine output can be due to gross hypovolaemia but may also indicate that the catheter is blocked or urine is leaking into the abdomen through a ruptured bladder or ureter.

Urine output may be artificially high in the first few hours after injury due to the diuretic effect of alcohol. A normal urine output does not exclude the diagnosis of hypovolaemia.

It is customary to measure urine output hourly. An output of 1 ml/kg body weight/hour normally indicates excellent renal perfusion. Volumes of 0.5 ml/kg/hour are acceptable. During resuscitation, it is often more helpful to make measurements at quarter hourly intervals. The absolute volumes obtained are small and may not truly reflect the actual output but it is often possible to detect trends which, when interpreted in the light of other monitoring parameters, are clinically helpful.

**Level of consciousness**.　During life-saving resuscitation, the critical level of unconsciousness occurs when the patient is unable to maintain and protect his airway. As resuscitation commences, a simple evaluation of the conscious level such as the AVPU method (Table 1.2.5) is all that is necessary. Using the AVPU method, patients in category U are certain to have airway and breathing problems. Those in category P are at significant risk while those in categories V and A are unlikely to need airway and breathing support.

As resuscitation proceeds, a more detailed method of monitoring conscious level is helpful. The Glasgow Coma Scale is widely used (Table 1.2.6). It was designed for use

**Table 1.2.5 AVPU method of assessing conscious level**

| | |
|---|---|
| A | *A*lert |
| V | Responds to *V*ocal stimuli |
| P | Responds to *P*ainful stimuli |
| U | *U*nresponsive |

**Table 1.2.6 Glasgow Coma Scale**

| | |
|---|---|
| *Eye-opening response* | |
| Spontaneous | 4 |
| To speech | 3 |
| To pain | 2 |
| None | 1 |
| | |
| *Best motor response* | |
| On command | 6 |
| Localizes in response to pain | 5 |
| Withdraws in response to pain | 4 |
| Abnormal flexion to pain | 3 |
| Extensor response to pain | 2 |
| No movement | 1 |
| | |
| *Verbal response* | |
| Orientated | 5 |
| Confused conversation | 4 |
| Inappropriate but recognizable words | 3 |
| Incomprehensible sounds | 2 |
| None | 1 |

with head injured patients but can be equally helpful for assessing altered consciousness from other causes such as hypoxia, hypovolaemia and hypothermia. Coma is defined as absent eye opening, inability to follow commands and absent word verbalization. This means that all patients with a Glasgow Coma Scale score of less than eight and most of those with a score of eight are in a coma. These patients are likely to have airway and breathing difficulties. Head injured patients with a score of nine or more are unlikely to have these difficulties unless there are other complicating factors such as a chest injury or severe haemorrhage. At the stage of resuscitation when the Glasgow Coma Scale score is being estimated, a single score is unlikely to alter clinical management because other more obvious signs of airway and breathing problems should already have been noted. The trend in Glasgow Coma Scale score can, however, be valuable for assessing the evolution of a head injury and the clinical response to therapeutic interventions.

**Central venous pressure**.   Central venous pressure measurement can be helpful in the later stages of life-saving resuscitation. Initially, all hypotensive patients should be assumed to be hypovolaemic. Fluids should be rapidly infused. Once the pulse rate and blood pressure have been restored to near normal, central venous pressure can be monitored to assist with the fine tuning of fluid administration and to help distinguish between the other causes of tachycardia and hypotension such as pain and fear. A raised central venous pressure in the presence of hypotension can confirm the diagnoses of cardiac tamponade or tension pneumothorax although the placement of a central venous pressure catheter for this purpose not only wastes valuable treatment time but is also unnecessary because distended neck veins should be clearly visible.

A central venous pressure of less than 5 cm $H_2O$ is indicative of hypovolaemia. It is common to find much higher values in hypovolaemic patients. A single central venous pressure measurement of greater than 5 cm $H_2O$ should never be accepted as a sign that the patient has an adequate blood volume. The trend in central venous pressure in response to repeated fluid challenges is a far better guide to the adequacy of the circulation. A persistent rise in central venous pressure indicates that the vascular space, *as it exists at the time of the measurement*, is well filled. Although the vascular space is well filled, the patient may still be maximally vasoconstricted and globally hypovolaemic.

It is tempting to use the central venous pressure catheter for the administration of resuscitation fluid. Most central venous pressure catheters are long and relatively small bore. This means that they are unsuitable for rapid fluid administration. Furthermore, fluid administration is interrupted every time a measurement is made. In the seriously injured patient it is unwise to rely on the central venous pressure catheter as a site of venous access for fluid administration although intermittent drug administration through the catheter is acceptable.

**Blood gas estimation**.   Blood gas estimation should not be helpful during life-saving resuscitation except as an indicator of the inadequacy of its management. Severe hypoxia or hypocarbia indicate that the patient has not been given 100% oxygen and that the signs of an inadequate airway or inadequate breathing have not been recognized. A metabolic acidosis is commonly present during resuscitation and may be a reflection of hypovolaemia and tissue hypoxia prior to admission. Correction with sodium bicarbonate is not indicated unless the arterial pH is less than 7.1. A metabolic acidosis will correct itself provided that airway, breathing and circulatory abnormalities are adequately treated. If the patient is fit enough, an arterial blood gas estimation taken after the patient has breathed room air for ten minutes can provide a useful baseline measurement which can be used to monitor future progress. No patient should be allowed to become hypoxic in order to obtain this measurement.

**Full blood count**.   A full blood count before resuscitation commences does not provide any useful information about the severity of blood loss. It is, however, useful as a baseline measurement as it may demonstrate pre-existing anaemia, infection or platelet insufficiency. Anaemia is a relatively common finding in Asian and elderly patients and usually reflects dietary insufficiency. Some young women with menorrhagia are also anaemic prior to their injury. Severe anaemia limits the oxygen-carrying capacity of the blood and can be an indication for the administration of blood sooner than would have normally been considered appropriate. Other parameters require careful interpretation. A raised white cell count, for example, reflects the presence of infection prior to admission but is also a common finding in head injured patients immediately after injury.

All severely injured patients must have blood taken for crossmatch. Blood for a full blood count can be taken at the same time. The investigation does not delay other life-saving activities and may be useful later on.

**Electrolyte and urea estimation**.   As with the full blood count, the estimation of urea and electrolytes serves only to provide a baseline measurement. In seriously injured patients, it is common to find that the serum potassium is low. This is probably related to the rises in glucose and insulin which occur as part of the stress response to injury and corrects itself within 24 hours. Active management is not required. The need for urea and electrolyte estimations on admission is debatable unless there is some reason to suspect a pre-existing abnormality such as the discovery of a prescription card for diuretics amongst the patient's possessions. Amongst the general population, unpredictable abnormalities of urea and electrolytes are rare.

**Blood sugar estimation**. Blood sugar is nearly always raised in seriously injured patients although the levels are rarely more than a few millimoles above normal. Treatment is not required. Although blood sugar is routinely measured, it is rarely clinically helpful unless the circumstances of the accident suggest that the onset of a diabetic coma due to hypoglycaemia or hyperglycaemia could have caused the accident and be a contibutory factor to the patient's existing clinical condition.

**End tidal carbon dioxide**. This measurement can be easily made if the patient requires intubation and ventilation. Used in conjunction with pulse oximetry, it is a helpful guide to the adequacy of ventilation prior to the insertion of an arterial line and the availability of serial blood gas estimations.

# Definitive management

# *The definitive diagnosis of injuries*

The life-saving resuscitation of an injured patient can be successfully achieved by the prompt recognition and treatment of the pathophysiological abnormalities caused by injury. During the later stages of resuscitation, a member of the resuscitation team will perform the secondary survey of the patient in order to diagnose all the injuries which are present. Following the secondary survey, radiological examination and other diagnostic techniques such as peritoneal lavage will be necessary. When all injuries have been diagnosed, their definitive management can begin.

During the secondary survey and while investigations are being performed, it is vital that the need for continuing oxygenation and fluid administration is recognized. The responsibilities of individual doctors during this time will depend on local circumstances and customs. The medical staff present during the admission of a seriously injured patient must work as a team and their skills be utilized to the patient's best advantage. In many hospitals it is customary for the anaesthetist to manage the airway and breathing while the A&E specialists in conjuction with their surgical colleagues manage fluid administration and the secondary survey. In addition to being skilled at airway management, anaesthetists also treat hypovolaemia and myocardial failure as part of their day-to-day work in the operating theatres and intensive care unit. It is helpful, therefore, if the anaesthetic member of the team monitors and contributes to the management of circulatory insufficiency too.

It is not normally customary for the anaestheist to be actively involved in the diagnostic process or in the surgical management of injuries. For the patient and the anaesthetist, there is some benefit if the anaesthetist has some knowledge of the diagnosis of injury and the pathophysiological effects of injury on oxygenation and blood loss. While it is perfectly possible for the anaesthetist to manage hypoxia and hypovolaemia with little or no knowledge of anything but the pathophysiological changes the injury has caused, an understanding of the known injuries will enable the anaesthetist to recognize pathophysiological changes which do not equate with known injuries. In particular, failure of resuscitative measures appropriate for diagnosed injuries should alert the anaesthetist to the possibility of other occult, and possibly life-threatening, injuries.

**History of injury.** The type of accident can give clues about the likely injuries. A classical example is the frontal impact road traffic accident when the patient is not restrained. Rapid deceleration occurs when a patient hits an immovable object such as the steering wheel or dash board. Significant thoracic injuries can occur. Aortic tears are a major risk because the arch of the aorta continues to move in the chest after impact but its root is fixed by mediastinal structures. Head injury, fractures of the cervical spine, abdominal injuries and posterior dislocation of the hips are also common as a result of this type of accident. If the patient is ejected from the vehicle, the risk of severe injury is increased by as much as three times.

Gun shot wounds produce a variable degree of injury depending on the velocity of the bullet, its shape and the proximity of the patient to the gun. A shot-gun, for example, fired at a distance of more than 12 metres normally damages skin and subcutaneous tissues but fired at point blank range causes extensive tissue damage and even death.

Stab wounds may cause minimal subcutaneous damage but if the implement is long, significant internal damage can occur. Even though the patient appears well and stable, serious injury should always be anticipated and the patient monitored closely until it can be ruled out.

**Examination**.    Systematic examination from head to toe will usually reveal most injuries. Look for bruising, lacerations, anatomical deformity, bleeding from orifices, asymmetry of the chest or limbs and marks caused by seat belts or tyres. Palpate for tenderness, surgical emphysema, boggy swellings and bony deformities not visible to the naked eye. Listen to the chest to assess the quality and quantity of air entry and to the abdomen for bowel sounds. Assess the level of consciousness using the Glasgow Coma Score (Table 1.2.6, p. 60).

Radiological examination of the chest and diagnostic peritoneal lavage may give additional information about chest and abdominal injuries respectively.

The information obtained will indicate the anatomical areas of injury. Used in addition to the information obtained during the resuscitation process, most injuries can be correctly diagnosed or at least suspected. After discussion with the surgeons, further investigations such as ultrasound, CT scanning, intravenous pyelography or laparotomy may be indicated.

## FURTHER READING

Grande, C.M. and Stene J.K. (1991). Mechanisms of injury: etiologies of trauma. In *Trauma Anesthesia* (Stene, J.K. and Grande, C.M., eds). Baltimore: Williams and Wilkins, pp. 37–63.

# *Estimating blood loss*

Blood loss after injury can vary immensely between patients. With the exception of loss from a major blood vessel, it is usually relatively slow but persistent. Bleeding from fracture sites may continue for 48 hours after injury. Fixation of fractures reduces the loss but does not necessarily stop it completely.

There are guidelines available for typical blood losses from a variety of injuries (Table 1.3.1). The amounts described represent the mean total loss from a given injury. Initial losses in the A&E department are likely to be smaller but these are only guidelines and there will always be exceptions.

External blood loss appears dramatic but is often less in volume than occult losses. Blood is similar in consistency to milk and recollection of the effects of spilling a bottle of milk may assist the anaesthetist in assessing the volume of blood

**Table 1.3.1 Guide to blood loss after injury**

| Injury | Blood loss (litres) |
| --- | --- |
| Fractured humerus | 0.5–1.0 |
| Foot or ankle fracture | 0.5–1.0 |
| Lower leg fracture | 0.5–1.5 |
| Femoral fracture | 1.5–3.0 |
| Pelvic fracture | 1.0–4.0 + |
| Rib fractures | 0.5–3.0 |
| Intra-abdominal injury | 1.0–6.0 + |
| Intrathoracic injury | 2.0–6.0 + |

loss onto the floor and bed linen! If dressings or swabs have been applied to wounds, estimations similar to those made in the operating theatre are useful.

The volume of blood loss into tissues is far more difficult to estimate. In addition, blood loss may be compounded by local oedema. Around a fractured femur, there may be as much as 2 litres of oedema fluid. As a rough guide, a swelling the size of a man's fist represents about 500 ml of blood and oedema. Swelling rarely occurs in this convenient manner. Large volumes can be lost into the thigh before a significant increase in circumference is measurable. Equally, an increase in abdominal girth may not be measurable until 3 or more litres of blood have been shed into the abdominal cavity. Measurement of thigh or abdominal girth is a poor guide to blood loss and is unhelpful as a guide to resuscitation.

Blood loss is most easily monitored and estimated using the parameters described previously (pp. 56–61). The clues described above are most helpful as comfirmatory, rather than diagnostic, evidence.

# *The significance of hypoxia during definitive management*

Even in the absence of chest injury or the pulmonary aspiration of stomach contents, hypoxia is common after injury. In a young fit man whose normal arterial oxygen tension is 14 kPa, it is not unusual to find an arterial oxygen tension of 10 kPa if supplemental oxygen is not provided. This is probably due to a combination of factors which include blood loss and pulmonary capillary obstruction due to microemboli and microthrombi. Values lower than 10 kPa indicate either profound hypovolaemia or a significant pulmonary insult.

## The significance of hypoxia

Arterial oxygen tension varies with age and with pre-existing lung disease. This can make it difficult to assess the significance of hypoxia. Table 1.3.2 shows the normal arterial oxygen tension at different ages. The degree of hypoxia due to pre-existing disease is almost impossible to assess. In the A&E department, it is probably safest to aim for a minimum arterial oxygen tension of 14 kPa in everyone. Higher levels are appropriate for hypotensive patients.

Apart from measuring the arterial oxygen tension to monitor the adequacy of oxygenation, it is also helpful to note trends. Controlled concentrations of oxygen can be given through an endotracheal tube but unfortunately, when oxygen is administered by face mask, it is impossible to be sure that the same concentration of oxygen is being administered as each blood sample is taken because even a minor malposition of the mask can permit air entrainment. When supplemental oxygen is given by mask, a decreasing trend in arterial oxygenation can only be regarded as significant if it is large. More significance can be attached to lesser changes in oxygenation if there are other signs of a deterioration in pulmonary function such as increasing respiratory rate, increasing confusion or increasing use of the accessory muscles of respiration. The anaesthetist should be alert to these changes because they may indicate significant un-

**Table 1.3.2 A guide to the effect of age on arterial oxygen tension**

| Age (years) | $PaO_2$ (kPa) |
| --- | --- |
| 10 | 14.0 |
| 20 | 13.0 |
| 30 | 12.0 |
| 40 | 11.5 |
| 50 | 11.0 |
| 60 | 10.5 |
| 70 | 9.5 |
| 80 | 9.0 |
| 90 | 8.5 |
| (Patient breathing room air) | |

diagnosed injuries such as a pneumothorax, pulmonary contusion, ruptures of the trachea or bronchi or diaphragmatic injury.

# Which fluid for transfusion?

There has been a long running debate concerning the best fluid for resuscitating trauma patients. Nobody disagrees that, ultimately, red cell loss must be replaced with red blood cells. Nor is there much argument about the type of red cells to be used. Whole blood is best if it is available but packed red cells are a satisfactory substitute if it is not.

The debate concerns whether crystalloid or colloid solutions are more appropriate prior to the administration of blood. Some of the confusion arises because of flaws in the original animal studies. Firstly, a variety of animals were used so that the results were not directly comparable. Secondly, the animal studies were performed under controlled conditions where haemorrhage was measured either as a controlled volume deficit or the animal was bled to a predetermined systolic blood pressure. Thirdly, often the animals were not injured. Consequently, none of the animal experimental work is truly representative of actual clinical conditions when the doctor is faced with a patient with a variety of injuries and a variable volume of blood loss causing a variable effect on blood pressure.

Studies on patients are also fraught with difficulty. It is possible to categorize injury severity using anatomical scores such as the Injury Severity Score, physiological scores such as the Revised Trauma Score or a combination of both such as TRISS. All these scores show reasonable correlation with the patient's eventual outcome but are not helpful when used for grouping patients according to the likely amount of blood loss. Early studies were also flawed because pulse and blood pressure were used as the end point for resuscitation and no allowance was made for the degree of vasoconstriction, and hence tissue hypoxia. More recent studies have used measurements of cardiac output and pulmonary artery occlusion pressure as the end point for resuscitation. Using these physiological end points, most studies have shown that there is very little to choose between isotonic crystalloid solutions and colloids in terms of either outcome or complication rate. Usually three times as much crystalloid solution as the volume of blood lost is required whereas isotonic colloid solutions can be used in volumes equal to the loss. In theory, therefore, unless a pulmonary artery flotation catheter is used for the resuscitation of every patient with major blood loss, the potential for error is greater with isotonic crystalloids because of the greater volumes used.

Other considerations such as cost and the risk of blood-borne infection are becoming increasingly important. While the former should not be allowed to compromise patient management, the latter is an important consideration which was neglected until the recent recognition of the autoimmune deficiency syndrome.

In practical terms, similar resuscitation protocols are used in nearly all centres, whether they profess to be crystalloid or colloid protagonists. Initially, up to 2 litres of isotonic crystalloid is given. Colloid is then given followed by uncrossmatched blood sufficient to maintain the haematocrit above 25%. When crossmatched blood is available, the haematocrit is maintained at 33% or above.

Recently it has been suggested that hypertonic saline solution may be a better alternative to other isotonic crystalloids. In small volumes, hypertonic saline is claimed to be safe but there is a real risk of sodium overload. The use of hypertonic saline is probably best regarded as a treatment which may find a place in resuscitation protocols in the not too distant future. It is too early yet to recommend it for routine use.

## FURTHER READING

Vincent, J-L. (1991). Fluids for resuscitation. *Brit. J. Anaesth.*, **67**, 185–193.
Shoemaker, W. C. and Kram W. B. (1988). Crystalloid and colloid therapy

resuscitation and subsequent ICU management. In *Clinical Anesthesiology* (Kox, W.J. and Gamble, J., eds) London : Baillière Tindall, vol. 2(3), pp. 509–544.

# *Monitoring the response to definitive management*

During the period of definitive management, it is vital that resuscitative measures continue and that the effects of these measures are closely monitored. The monitoring techniques used during resuscitation for life-threatening problems (pp. 54–55) are still helpful. At this stage, it is particularly important to note trends in monitoring parameters. The patient's condition should have stabilized and resuscitative measures should match continuing, but predictable, changes in the patient's condition. Acute airway problems, for example, will already have been dealt with. Nevertheless, some head injured patients may slowly develop cerebral oedema and, as their conscious level falls, may require airway protection. A patient with fractured ribs may suddenly develop a pneumothorax. Continued blood loss from fractures is normal. The possibility that problems such as these may develop must be anticipated and the patient's vital signs monitored accordingly.

During the period of definitive management, the initial flurry of activity which was necessary when the patient was admitted should have given way to a more sedate approach to management. Priorities for examination, investigation and treatment will be being decided. Amongst these priorities, will be the commencement of more sophisticated monitoring techniques. Now may be the time to insert a central venous pressure catheter if one has not already been sited. An in-dwelling arterial cannula will almost certainly be needed at some stage during the next few hours. Its placement at this stage will allow continuous display of the blood pressure, repeated sampling of blood for gas, acid base and, if necessary, haemoglobin and electrolyte estimations. Consideration should also be given to the need for a pulmonary artery flotation catheter for monitoring of cardiac output, pulmonary capillary wedge pressure, systemic vascular resistance and oxygen flux. There is no doubt that the measurements obtained from a pulmonary artery flotation catheter provide the most helpful and accurate information about the progress of resuscitation. The problem is that these catheters are associated with a significant number of complications, the most serious of which are pulmonary artery rupture and pulmonary infarction. The risks of inserting the catheter must be balanced against the benefits obtained from the measurements made. In young, fit adults with uncomplicated blood loss, monitoring of the central venous pressure and urine output is probably all that is required particularly if the urine output has never been reduced. Maintenance of a normal urine output implies that compensatory vasoconstriction has never been maximal and that the degree of tissue hypoxia resulting from blood loss is unlikely to have been severe. There may be a case for using a pulmonary artery flotation catheter for young fit patients if blood loss is likely to be heavy and prolonged. This sort of situation can be expected if patients have suffered severe pelvic fractures with diastasis of the symphysis pubis or if the patient has a ruptured liver or major intrathoracic blood vessel injury. In the presence of these injuries, the anaesthetist must consider whether the catheter is better placed in the A&E department where sterile conditions are not all that easy to maintain or whether it would be better to wait until the patient can be transferred to the operating theatre or intensive care unit. The decision will depend on how long the patient is expected to remain in the A&E department, the urgency with which the measurements it gives are required and on local circumstances and protocols. In many A&E departments, cardiac output monitoring is not routinely available. If this is the case, it is usually better to move the patient to the monitoring equipment rather than the monitoring equipment to the patient. The patient may, however, need to remain in the A&E or Radiology department for completion of the radiological examination. The need for cardiac output monitoring implies that the patient is unstable and severely ill. The risks of not monitoring the patient in this manner must be weighed against the risks of not completing the radiological or other examinations at this stage.

The use of a pulmonary artery flotation catheter is more clearly indicated when severe haemorrhage is occurring and there is also evidence of damage to the heart or lungs. The measurement of central venous pressure is not helpful in this situation and effective resuscitation depends on the measurement of pulmonary capillary wedge pressure, cardiac output and oxygen flux to optimize the combined use of fluid and inotropic drugs. Use of a pulmonary artery flotation catheter is essential to monitor the effects of fluid replacement and to avoid fluid overload. It is also essential for the diagnosis and treatment of myocardial failure.

The formation of interstitial oedema is inevitable if the lungs have been injured (p. 97). Fluid overload increases the severity of the oedema. Under-transfusion reduces oedema formation but may increase tissue hypoxia in a patient who is already at risk because of a severe pulmonary injury. The concurrence of significant haemorrhage and severe pulmonary injury is usually a compelling indication for the use of a pulmonary artery flotation catheter.

# Reassessment of the patient after definitive management

With a basic knowledge of the normal degree of hypovolaemia and hypoxia associated with identified injuries and regular monitoring of the progress of resuscitation and treatment, the anaesthetist should be able to detect a mismatch between the patient's requirements as indicated by the parameters being monitored and his requirements as estimated from the known injuries. The patient must be re-examined and investigated for other undiagnosed injuries. These are most likely to be intra-abdominal or intra-thoracic but the patient should be examined again from head to toe and an explanation for the discrepancy sought. Usually, unexpectedly severe hypoxia is due to an undetected injury to the respiratory tract. Excessive haemorrhage from intra-thoracic and intra-abdominal organs must be excluded but can also be due to extensive soft tissue bruising, large scalp lacerations or even from a fracture of the nasal bones. During the initial resuscitation and examination, this type of injury is often dismissed as trivial and forgotten. It is, however, possible for a patient to lose over 50% of his blood volume from this type of 'minor' injury. Usually excessive blood loss is suspected because the pulse and blood pressure fail to respond to intravenous fluids and usually this supposition is correct. Other causes of hypotension must always be considered, especially if a source of bleeding cannot be found. Cardiac tamponade and tension pneumothorax are important causes of hypotension that may become apparent at this time.

Even if resuscitation is proceeding as expected, it is essential to reassess the patient after as much definitive treatment as is possible has been carried out in the A&E department. It is unlikely, but possible, that other major injuries will be detected. It is probable that other minor injuries, such as fractures of the metacarpals or small lacerations, will be found. These injuries are not life threatening and may heal in the absence of treatment. Prompt treatment may, however, ensure a better outcome. Often, patients who survive severe major injuries will later complain of complications from minor injuries. To the doctor, these complications may appear trivial in the light of the patient's uncomplicated recovery from other major injuries. To the patient, who often has no memory of the time during recovery from his major injuries, these complications are important.

# Provision of analgesia during definitive management

Pain relief is an important part of the definitive management of the severely injured patient. It is often relegated to the bottom of the list of priorities because of fear of masking clinical signs, fear of causing hypotension and because it is not essential to the recovery of the patient. From the patient's perspective, pain is one of the most feared aspects of illness and injury, and its prompt treatment is greeted with gratitude. From the doctor's point of view, provided that the method of pain relief is chosen with care, clinical signs will not be masked to the extent that injuries are missed, hypotension is not inevitable and the vasoconstriction, hypertension and tachycardia secondary to pain will be relieved. This means that all of these signs can be used more readily to assess the extent of hypovolaemia. Furthermore, a patient whose pain is tolerable is easier to examine and is likely to be more cooperative during the insertion of invasive monitoring devices and with other methods of treatment.

The choice of analgesic agent depends on the nature and severity of the pain and on the interaction of the agent and injuries. It is sometimes appropriate to use more than one method of analgesia, particularly if the patient has multiple injuries.

**Entonox**. A 50/50 mixture of oxygen and nitrous oxide administered correctly through a tightly fitting face mask is said to provide analgesia equivalent to 10 mg morphine given intramuscularly. Entonox rarely causes unconsciousness in normovolaemic patients but can do so in hypovolaemic patients. This is not a problem if the patient self-administers Entonox because, as the patient falls asleep, the mask drops away from the face. Many severely injured patients are unable to hold the mask for themselves. The anaesthetist may have to administer the Entonox and must monitor the patient's level of consciousness and analgesia. Entonox is safe because it does not cause significant alterations in blood pressure, respiration or intracranial pressure. It can also be stopped at will and the pain will rapidly return if the surgeons require it to aid diagnosis. Because of the greater solubility of nitrous oxide compared to nitrogen, Entonox increases the volume of gas in closed spaces. It may convert a simple pneumothorax to a tension pneumothorax, increase the volume of gas in the bowels or raise intracranial pressure if air is present within the skull. None of these problems are common and provided that the anaesthetist is aware of its potential dangers, Entonox can be given to all injured patients.

In practice, there are only four limitations to its use in the A&E department. The amount of analgesia is often insufficient for young men with severe pain, the inspired oxygen concentration is limited to 50% and injuries which alter the facial contour make make it difficult to administer. Because the cylinders are bulky, it is unusual to find more than one available in each department. This limits the number of patients who can be treated.

**Local anaesthetic techniques**.  These techniques are useful for the relief of pain due to limb injuries. Almost any peripheral nerve can be blocked. The choice depends on the type of injury. Commonly, a femoral nerve block is the best form of analgesia for femoral shaft fractures and if administered prior to the application of traction or a splint can render these procedures almost painless. The pain from extensive injuries to the arm can be treated with a brachial plexus block. If there is damage to the blood vessels, the sympathetic blockade and vasodilatation can be helpful when the vessels are subsequently repaired. Use of peripheral nerve blocks does make clinical evaluation of nerve injuries difficult so this form of analgesia should be withheld until the surgeons have completed their assessment of the injury.

Epidural anaesthesia at lumbar level is one of the best forms of pain relief for pelvic fractures and can diminish the amount of bleeding. Similarly, thoracic epidural anaesthesia is helpful for thoracic injuries. In the A&E department,

caution is required. Profound falls in blood pressure secondary to vasodilatation may occur if the patient's blood volume
has not been completely restored and vasoconstriction reversed. Accidental dural tap is hazardous in the head injured
patient with raised intracranial pressure because it may
precipitate coning of the brain stem through the foramen
magnum. Epidural anaesthesia should not be administered in
the presence of clotting abnormalities but this is rarely a
problem in the A&E department. Finally, aseptic technique
is essential during insertion. The choice of analgesic agent is
between a local anaesthetic, a preservative free opiate or a
combination of the two. In the A&E department, it is
probably better to use an opiate which causes less fall in bood
pressure but often the pain relief is not as effective as that
provided by a local anaesthetic agent or combination of
drugs.

**Opiate analgesia**. The opiate group of analgesics provide
potent pain relief. They can be administered by the oral,
intramuscular, intravenous or intrathecal routes. The intravenous route is the most useful because a bolus dose can be
titrated against the patient's individual requirement and can
be followed up with an infusion which maintains constant
blood levels and prevents breakthrough pain which is often
experienced if bolus doses are inappropriately spaced.

The opiate analgesics are claimed to have many disadvantages which relate to their side-effects. The risk of respiratory
depression is often quoted as a reason for withholding or
giving inadequate doses, particularly if the patient is already
in respiratory distress. If the distress is due to pain, an opiate
will often improve respiratory function. Furthermore, the
risk of respiratory depression is greatly reduced if the dose is
administered intravenously and is titrated against the
patient's perception of pain when he is undisturbed. Opiates
are also said to reduce blood pressure. This is true. The fall
in blood pressure is due partly to histamine release but
mainly due to the reversal of vasoconstriction caused by
pain. If hypotension is anticipated and blood is transfused to
fill the expanded vascular space, significant falls in blood
pressure can be prevented.

Opiate analgesics are frequently withheld for fear of masking clinical signs. Pain is useful as an easily detectable clue that an injury has been sustained in a particular area, but once its presence has been noted, the diagnosis of injury can be made by other means. It is, therefore, reasonable to withhold opiate analgesia until the secondary survey has been completed but not for any longer. There are a few instances when the presence of increasing pain is an important clinical sign. Ischaemic limb pain due to arterial injury or compartment syndrome should not be ignored but is usually manifest as an increasing need for analgesia. The severity of pain is such that the original prescribed dose of opiate becomes insufficient. Whereas continuing complaints of pain from an untreated patient may be ignored because they are expected, a change in the level of pain in a previously pain-free patient may actually draw attention to a change in the patient's condition.

The administration of opiate analgesics to head injured patients is contentious. It is usually said that opiates are contraindicated in this situation because they may mask pupillary changes or alter conscious level. In practice, it is unusual for opiates to prevent dilatation of the pupil in response to the development of an intracranial haematoma. If the initial dose is carefully titrated so that the patient remains conscious, any change in conscious level can safely be attributed to factors other than the opiate. The main difficulty encountered in administering opiates to head injured patients is not in the side-effects of the opiates but in the tendency of inexperienced medical and nursing staff to blame changes in the patient's clinical condition on the opiates. If staff can be trained to recognize the normal changes induced by carefully titrated doses of opiates, it should be possible for them to recognize deteriorations in the patient's clinical condition which are consistent with rises in intracranial pressure. If this is not possible, it is safer to give codeine phosphate to head injured patients but this may mean that adequate analgesia is impossible to achieve. The administration of opiates by the intrathecal route is contraindicated in head injured patients because, if intracranial pressure is raised, insertion of a needle into the lumbar subarachnoid space may cause leakage of cerebrospinal fluid, a fall in pressure and coning of the brain stem through the foramen magnum.

**Non-steroidal anti-inflammatory agents**. Drugs in this group are particularly effective for pain due to soft tissue injuries. They are rarely appropriate for patients with major trauma. There is, however, a small body of evidence suggesting that non-steroidal anti-inflammatory agents used in conjunction with opiates may provide better pain relief than that provided by either type of drug used alone. Furthermore, effective analgesia using this drug combination can be achieved using lower than normal doses of each type of drug. This has obvious advantages if side-effects are a potential management problem.

**FURTHER READING**

Zenz, M., Panhans, C., Niesel, H. Chr. and Kreuscher, H. (1988). *Regional Anaesthesia*. London : Wolfe Medical Publications Ltd.
Fields, H.L. (1987). *Pain*. New York: McGraw-Hill.

# *The use of sedative drugs during definitive management*

It is not unusual for severely injured patients to be agitated, aggressive, uncooperative, or generally disruptive in the A&E department. This can make diagnosis and treatment extremely difficult. The patient who thrashes about the bed is at risk of further injury. He may also be at increased risk if diagnosis is delayed and treatment cannot be given promptly. It is tempting to sedate the agitated patient. There are many possible reasons for agitation and aggression in the severely injured patient. These are listed in Table 1.3.3. When, and

**Table 1.3.3 Causes of confusion and agitation in the injured patient**

| | |
|---|---|
| Hypoxia | Alcohol abuse |
| Hypovolaemia | Drug abuse |
| Head injury | |
| Anxiety | Psychosis |
| Pain | |

only when, all possible causes of agitation and confusion have been considered and treated, the administration of a sedative drug may be considered.

The treatment of most of the causes of confusion and aggression is considered elsewhere. Agitation due to alcoholic intoxication and head injury are difficult to treat. In the case of a head injury, increasing conscious level associated with increasing agitation is usually a sign of recovery. Very rarely, increasing agitation is the first sign of a subdural haematoma. As such, the increasing level of agitation is a useful diagnostic sign and it is preferable to physically restrain the patient, rather than to sedate him. Alcoholic intoxication is often associated with head injury. For the reasons given previously, restraint is usually the treatment of choice. If it is certain that a head injury has not been sustained, the use of a small dose of benzodiazepine or chlormethiazole is acceptable.

Sometimes patients become agitated and uncooperative because of the psychological shock of the accident, fear of what the eventual outcome of their injuries will be or because they are worried about relations or friends who were also involved in the accident. Usually, reassurance from the nursing staff or doctors is all that is required but it takes a long time for the information imparted to be retained. Repeated reassurances are necessary and should form part of the patient's definitive care. If the patient has a true and frightening understanding of his or his relative's injuries, a small dose of an anxiolytic such as Diazemuls® or midazolam may be helpful. In this situation the anxiolytic may also reduce the dose of analgesic agents required because anxiety can reduce the pain threshhold.

Rarely, the acute onset of a psychotic state has precipitated a suicide attempt. Patients under the influence of hallucinogenic drugs may attempt to fly or perform other feats which are not within the human capability. For these patients, the use of sedatives may be positively indicated as part of the definitive management of the patient's mental disturbance.

# Emergency surgery in the resuscitation room

Rarely, surgery in the resuscitation room may prove life-saving. Emergency surgery is defined as 'surgery which is required within an hour of admission and which is performed concurrently with resuscitation'. In fact, the surgery should be regarded as part of the resuscitation process. There are very few indications for emergency surgery. These are listed in Table 1.3.4. The operations involved are tracheostomy, thoracotomy, burr holes and laparotomy.

Emergency surgery and anaesthesia require close cooperation between the anaesthetist and the surgeon. The risks of performing surgery in a non-sterile environment which is not

**Table 1.3.4 Indications for surgery in the resuscitation room**

1. Airway obstruction or disruption which is not amenable to treatment by endotracheal intubation
2. Massive haemorrhage when blood pressure cannot be maintained by rapid transfusion
3. Rapidly enlarging intracranial haematoma
4. Cardiorespiratory arrest unresponsive to external cardiac massage

as well equipped as an operating theatre must be balanced against the risks of delaying surgery until the patient can be transferred to a fully equipped operating theatre. Patients who cannot be transferred to an operating theatre are usually moribund, or have suffered a cardiorespiratory arrest, and are certain to die if surgery is not performed immediately. The risks are, therefore, well worth taking if life can be preserved. Sadly, even if surgery is performed rapidly, most patients undergoing surgery in the resuscitation room do not survive.

# Anaesthesia for surgery in the resuscitation room

## GENERAL CONSIDERATIONS

Patients requiring surgery in the resuscitation room are moribund and usually deeply unconscious. Initial anaesthetic management is, therefore, related to continuing resuscitation of the airway, breathing and circulation. Endotracheal intubation, the administration of high concentrations of oxygen, controlled mechanical ventilation, insertion of large bore intravenous cannulae and administration of blood continue to be high priorities, just as they are when the patient is admitted. Close monitoring of arterial oxygenation and the patient's cardiovascular status are vital. Initially, the only anaesthetic drugs which are required are muscle relaxants. The relaxant should be chosen according to its haemodynamic effects (see Table 1.3.5). It is important to maintain normal blood pressure in the head injured patient so relaxants with minimal effects on the circulation should be chosen. If the patient is hypovolaemic, many anaesthetists choose pancuronium because it raises blood pressure.

As the patient's condition improves, there may be a need to administer analgesic or anaesthetic agents in order to

**Table 1.3.5 The haemodynamic effects of anaesthetic agents**

|                | Dose (mg/kg) | HR  | MABP | CO  | SVR |
|----------------|--------------|-----|------|-----|-----|
| Etomidate      | 0.45         | +   | −    | −   | −   |
| Ketamine       | 2.0          | +++ | +++  | +++ | 0   |
| Propofol       | 1.6          | −   | −−−  | −−− | −−  |
| Thiopentone    | 4.0          | 0   | −−   | −−  | −   |
| Midazolam      | 0.25         | 0   | −    | −   | −−  |
| Nitrous oxide  | 40%          | −−  | −    | −−  | +++ |
| Enflurane      | 2%           | ++  | −−−  | −−  | −−  |
| Halothane      | 1%           | +   | −−−  | −−  | −   |
| Isoflurane     | 1%           | ++  | −−−  | 0   | −−− |
| Suxamethonium  | 1.0          | +   | ++   | ?   | ?   |
| Alcuronium     | 0.15         | +   | 0    | +   | −   |
| Atracurium     | 0.4          | +   | −    | +   | −   |
| d-Tubocurarine | 0.4          | +   | −−−  | −   | −−− |
| Pancuronium    | 0.07         | ++  | ++   | ++  | −   |
| Vecuronium     | 0.28         | 0   | −    | +   | −−  |
| Alfentanyl     | 0.125        | 0   | −    | −   | −   |
| Fentanyl       | 0.075        | −   | −    | −−  | −   |
| Morphine       | 1.0          | −   | −    | 0   | 0   |
| Pethidine      | 1.0          | ++  | 0    | ++  | −   |
| Atropine       | 0.6/70 kg    | ++  | +    | ++  | −−  |

N.B. Doses for similar drugs are not equipotent and the effect may be different if two or more drugs are used in combination.
Based on Woerlee, G.M. (1988). *Common Perioperative Problems and the Anaesthetist.* Dordrecht: Kluwer Academic Publishers.

ensure that the patient is unconscious throughout the procedure. Again, the choice of agent depends on the patient's
haemodynamic stability. Ketamine, administered as an infusion, can be a useful method of anaesthesia for hypovolaemic
patients because it normally increases cardiac output and
blood pressure. The rise in blood pressure is associated with
a rise in intracranial pressure. Head injury is, therefore, a
contraindication to the use of ketamine. It is also useful in
haemodynamically stable patients with compromised breathing because it does not normally depress respiration or
obtund protective airway reflexes. It is also an excellent
analgesic agent. Alternatively, high dose fentanyl by infusion
is sometimes recommended because it has no deleterious

effects on cardiac output and blood pressure. In the presence of continued bleeding, titrating of the dose of intravenous agents can be difficult. Nitrous oxide, supplemented by a volatile agent, may be a better option although vasodilatation and depression of myocardial contractility are significant problems in the hypovolaemic patient. Rises in intrathoracic pressure caused by positive pressure ventilation may cause hypotension in hypovolaemic patients. The ventilator should be set so that the tidal and minute volumes delivered are the minimum required to produce adequate arterial oxygenation and carbon dioxide removal.

**Ruptured trachea or bronchus**.   If a thoracotomy is required for major tears or total disruption of the trachea or major airways, the anaesthetist must be prepared to intubate the airway at the level of the injury after the chest has been opened. This means that endotracheal tubes of varying sizes must be instantly available on the surgical instrument trolley and must have compatible connections with the equipment to be used for ventilation. The anaesthetist must be prepared to maintain one lung anaesthesia and oxygenation while the defect is repaired.

**Intracranial haematoma**.   The management of the head injured patient who has developed a subdural or extradural haematoma is rather different from the management of other patients requiring emergency surgery in the resuscitation room. If surgery is truly urgent enough to be performed in the resuscitation room, it can be assumed that the intracranial pressure is very high. Every attempt must be made to lower the intracranial pressure as quickly as possible. Measures described in Table 1.4.1 (p. 89) should be employed. Although the patient will be deeply unconscious, there is some merit in administering a sleep dose of an induction agent such as thiopentone, etomidate or propofol together with suxamethonium. These agents will reduce the hypertensive response to intubation and prevent a rise in intracranial pressure.

# Specific injuries of importance to the anaesthetist

# *Head injury*

The anaesthetist is likely to be involved in the care of the most seriously head injured patients whose initial presentation includes airway difficulties. Persistent unconsciousness from the time of the accident is due to primary brain injury. Most patients wake up quite quickly but a few with severe brain injury may remain unconscious for some time. This type of patient frequently develops cerebral oedema which causes a further decrease in conscious level. The outcome after severe head injury is often poor and, provided cerebral swelling is controlled, depends on the severity of the primary brain injury. The eventual outcome may be far worse if secondary brain injury occurs due to hypoxia and hypovolaemia. All severely head injured patients must be closely monitored for signs of airway, breathing and circulatory abnormalities and corrective action must be prompt.

Approximately 20% of patients with relatively minor primary brain injury and a skull fracture develop an extradural or subdural haematoma. These patients characteristically suffer a short period of unconsciousness followed by a lucid interval before lapsing into a deep coma. Surgical removal of the haematoma is essential. Mannitol given in a dose of 0.5 mg/kg/body weight over one half hour may temporarily reduce the volume of the intracranial contents and thus intracranial pressure. This is only a temporary measure but may buy enough time to allow a CT scan to be performed prior to surgery. A CT scan is helpful because it confirms the diagnosis and permits accurate localization of the haematoma. Patients who have developed an intracranial haematoma acutely usually require endotracheal intubation to protect their airway. Controlled mechanical ventilation is also helpful to lower the arterial carbon dioxide tension to between 3.5 and 4.0 kPa. At this level, the cerebral blood vessels are vasoconstricted to the minimum size consistent with adequate cerebral blood flow and oxygenation.

**Raised intracranial pressure**.   Raised intracranial pressure is known to be associated with a high mortality rate in head injured patients but it is often hard to identify how much of the mortality rate is due to the primary brain injury and how much is due to the additional effects of the oedema and hyperaemia which occur secondary to the brain injury.

Normally, cerebral blood flow is autoregulated in the mean arterial pressure range of 60 to 130 mmHg. Outside this pressure range, cerebral blood flow is proportional to the mean arterial pressure. Autoregulation is lost in damaged areas of brain in which case cerebral blood flow is a function of cerebral perfusion pressure which is calculated by subtracting intracranial pressure from mean arterial blood pressure. A cerebral perfusion pressure of at least 30 mmHg is essential to maintain normal cerebral blood flow.

Cerebral blood flow is also proportional to arterial carbon dioxide tension in the range of 2.7 to 6.7 kPa. Cerebral vasoconstriction caused by acute hypocarbia can produce dramatic falls in intracranial pressure but over a period of days the cerebral blood flow will adjust to a persistently low level of arterial carbon dioxide and will return to pre-injury levels. Cerebral blood flow does not alter in response to arterial oxygenation until the arterial oxygen tension falls below 6.7 kPa when vasodilatation occurs.

In the head injured patient with raised intracranial pressure, the relationship between cerebral blood flow, intracranial pressure and blood pressure is unpredictable and there are regional differences between areas of normal and abnormal brain. It has never been clearly demonstrated that measures to reduce intracranial pressure have a beneficial effect on outcome. This may be because it is so difficult to distinguish between patients with coma due mainly to primary brain injury and those with coma due mainly to reversible rises in intracranial pressure. In spite of the current lack of positive evidence in favour of controlling intracranial pressure, it is wise to make every attempt to control intracranial pressure. The methods available are shown in Table 1.4.1. If measures to control intracranial pressure do improve outcome, it is logical that they be started as promptly as possible in the A&E department rather than waiting until the patient is admitted to the Intensive Care Unit.

**Intracranial haematoma**. The characteristic features of a developing intracranial haematoma are a lucid interval followed by decreasing conscious level, the development of localizing neurological signs and, latterly, pupillary dilatation on the contralateral side to the haematoma. Some severely head injured patients do not have a lucid interval before a haematoma develops. Frequently, these patients have required airway maintenance since the time of admission. If the patient requires paralysis and mechanical ventilation, the only clinical sign of a developing haematoma may be a change in the size of the pupils. The anaesthetist can do very little in the A&E department to assist the surgeon in making the diagnosis. Maintenance of the airway by manual methods for a brief period so that the surgeon can make a rapid

**Table 1.4.1 Methods of controlling intracranial pressure**

---

*Basic measures*
Clear the airway
Give oxygen
Establish effective ventilation
Head up tilt
Straighten neck
Avoid tight tapes around neck
CT scan to exclude a surgically remediable haematoma

*If ventilated*
Maintain $PaCO_2$ between 3.5 and 4.0 kPa
Maintain minimum mean intrathoracic pressure compatible with adequate
   oxygenation and control of $PaCO_2$

*If raised intracranial pressure suspected or positively diagnosed*
Sedation and analgesia to control blood pressure and heart rate
Restrict crystalloid fluid volume to 50 ml/hr
Mannitol 0.5 mg/kg IV *or* Frusemide 40 mg IV

*If raised intracranial pressure has been positively diagnosed and the measures
listed above do not provide adequate control consider*
Thiopentone infusion
Propofol infusion
Hypothermia

---

neurological assessment of the patient before paralysis with
muscle relaxants can be helpful. Use of a short-acting muscle
relaxant such as atracurium or vecuronium is helpful because
the patient can be intermittently reversed with neostigmine
and atropine to permit reassessment of the patient's neurological status. It is also important that the patient is monitored
closely. Changes in pulse rate, blood pressure and cardiac
rhythm may indicate that the intracranial pressure is rising
but do not distinguish between raised pressure due to a space
occupying lesion and raised pressure due to cerebal oedema
or hyperaemia. Reversal and examination of the patient may
be of assistance but CT scanning is the best method of
making a positive diagnosis.

Very rarely, a patient who is regaining consciousness and
who becomes increasingly agitated is developing an intra-

cranial haematoma. It is impossible to distinguish these patients from those making a normal recovery unless intracranial pressure is measured or a CT scan is performed. Sedatives should never be given to agitated, head injured patients unless intracranial bleeding can be positively excluded as the sedative may decrease the conscious level and mask the eventual, inevitable decrease in conscious level caused by the haematoma. The agitated patient may be a danger to himself or others. If sedation cannot be given safely, physical restraint may be necessary.

**Neurogenic pulmonary oedema**. Occasionally, the primary head injury causes massive sympathetic stimulation. This is manifest clinically as intense peripheral vasoconstriction and neurogenic pulmonary oedema. The pulmonary oedema can be copious, may be heavily blood stained, and can cause severe hypoxia. It may be sudden in onset and if the patient is not already intubated can make this procedure difficult because the larynx is obscured by a constant flow of oedema fluid. It may be necessary to intubate blindly, aiming for the area where exhaled gases cause frothing of the oedema fluid. Treatment is difficult. Mechanical ventilation with 100% oxygen and positive end expiratory pressure can help, but the latter raises intrathoracic pressure and may reduce venous return and increase intracranial pressure. Sympathetic blockade may be helpful but the drug used must be chosen with care because a fall in blood pressure may reduce cerebral blood flow and dilatation of the cerebral vasculature may raise intracranial pressure. Of all the drugs available, intravenous labetalol used in tiny incremental doses of 1 to 2 mg is probably the best choice.

**Multiple injuries**. Head injured patients frequently have other injuries. Because the patient is unconscious, he cannot complain of pain and these injuries may be missed unless they are actively sought. The importance of close monitoring to ensure adequate oxygenation and fluid replacement cannot be overemphasized. The injuries most likely to be missed are those in the chest and abdomen. These are the injuries which cause hypoxia and major haemorrhage. All head injured patients benefit from repeated examination of the chest and, if indicated, serial chest X-rays. Diagnostic peritoneal lavage is indicated in all head injured patients whose expected blood loss does not match their actual fluid requirement.

**Anaesthesia for head injured patients in the A&E department.** Anaesthesia may be required prior to emergency surgery for the evacuation of an intracranial haematoma or to facilitate endotracheal intubation for protection of the airway or control of arterial carbon dioxide tension. The key features of anaesthesia for head injured patients are protection of the airway, the maintenance of adequate oxygenation, the maintenance of a stable blood pressure and the avoidance of drugs and manoeuvres which may raise intracranial pressure. All patients must be resuscitated prior to the induction of anaesthesia. The induction and intubation must be as smooth as possible with minimal alterations in blood pressure. This may be achieved by administering topical lignocaine or intravenous fentanyl prior to laryngoscopy. The patient must always be ventilated. Anaesthesia with spontaneous respiration is associated with an inevitable rise in arterial carbon dioxide which will dilate blood vessels and raise intracranial pressure. The anaesthetic agents used should be chosen for their beneficial effects on intracranial pressure ( Table 1.4.2) and their lack of deleterious effect on haemodynamic stability (Table 1.3.5, p. 84).

## FURTHER READING

North, B. and Reilly, P. (1990). *Raised Intracranial Pressure – a Clinical Guide*. Oxford: Heinemann Medical Books.
Jennett, B. and Teasdale, G. (1982). *Management of Head Injuries*. Philadelphia: F. A. Davis Co.

**Table 1.4.2 The effects of anaesthetic drugs on intracranial pressure and cerebral perfusion pressure**

|  | Intracranial pressure | Cerebral perfusion pressure |
|---|---|---|
| Etomidate | − − − | 0/− |
| Ketamine | + + + | − − − |
| Propofol | − − − | 0/− |
| Thiopentone | − − − | − − |
| Fentanyl | − | − |
| Morphine | − | − |
| Volatile agents (constant PaCO$_2$) | + + + | − − − |

# Cervical spine injury

Patients with cervical spine injury may be divided into four main categories. These are:

1. Patients with a cervical spine fracture but no neurological deficit and no other injuries.
2. Patients with cervical spine fracture, no neurological deficit and other injuries.
3. Patients with cervical spine fracture, neurological deficit and no other injury.
4. Patients with cervical spine fracture, neurological deficit and other injuries.

It is important to differentiate between the groups because their clinical signs and management are completely different. Group 1, for example, are unlikely to need the assistance of the anaesthetist and their management consists of immobilizing the spine. Often skull traction is applied. Infiltration of the skin with local anaesthetic is all that is required. Group 2 patients may require the resuscitative measures described in preceding sections to maintain adequate oxygenation and ventilation. The anaesthetist's main concern is to avoid damage to the spinal cord during intubation. Group 3 and Group 4 patients have specific pathophysiological alterations secondary to the spinal cord injury and subsequent neurological deficit. It is important that these changes are recognized and managed correctly and that they are distinguished from the pathophysiological changes due to other injuries. As with head injury, spinal cord injury has three distinct components. These are primary cord injury which does not recover, oedema around the area of injury which may recover and secondary cord damage due to hypoxia and hypovolaemia.

**Pathphysiological changes due to spinal cord injury**. Loss of neurological control has many effects which include inadequate breathing, cardiovascular instability due to vasodilatation and damage to the cardiac ganglia, susceptibility to skin damage and pressure sores, loss of normal bowel tone and the onset of paralytic ileus, loss of bladder control, retention of urine and autonomic hyperreflexia. The severity of these changes depends on the level of the initial spinal cord injury and the subsequent extent of spinal cord oedema and tissue hypoxia. Noradrenaline may be released at the site of injury and cause localized vasoconstriction.

**Management of the pathophysiological effects of spinal cord injury**. The approach should be the same as for all other injuries; namely, attention to airway, breathing and circulation. The airway is normally intact. The adequacy of respiration depends on the level of the injury. Patients with lesions at or below C4 usually do not have difficulty breathing initially because, even though the intercostal muscles are paralysed, adequate gas exchange can be achieved with the use of the diaphragm and accessory muscles of respiration such as the scalenes, sternocleidomastoids and trapezii. These patients require close monitoring because breathing may subsequently become inadequate due to muscle fatigue or sputum retention.

Patients with lesions above C3 depend entirely on their accessory muscles for ventilation. The respiratory movements produced may be sufficient to allow patients to reach hospital alive but respiratory assistance is often necessary shortly after admission.

The decision to intubate a patient with a spinal cord injury is made on clinical grounds. Inadequate respiration sufficient to cause hypoxia is a good indication for intubation on admission. Other patients should be monitored closely and intubated if there is a definite downward trend in respiratory monitoring parameters.

The blood pressure is usually low due to loss of sympathetic tone and massive vasodilatation below the level of the injury. Patients with spinal cord injury tend to maintain a below average blood pressure. Transfusion of crystalloid or colloid solutions to restore the blood pressure to a systolic pressure of 90 to 100 mmHg is usually sufficient and the volume required is rarely more than 2 litres. Pulmonary oedema is easily precipitated by volume overload. It may also occur in the presence of normovolaemia. The reason for this is not well understood but it could be related to a massive sympathetic discharge similar to that which occurs after a severe head injury. Transfusion should be limited to the volume required to maintain a urine output of 50 ml/hour. In the early stages of management, an indwelling catheter can be used to monitor urine output. Intermittent catheterization can be commenced when the patient has been stabilized. Central venous pressure monitoring is helpful in the A&E department. If there is doubt about the adequacy of tissue perfusion a pulmonary artery flotation catheter may be used but is rarely required in the early stages of resuscitation. Sometimes the blood pressure is adversely affected by dysrhythmias due to the loss of autonomic control of the cardiac rhythm. Treatment depends on the nature of the rhythm. Bradycardia, which responds to atropine, is by far the commonest dysrhythmia.

Although sympathetic activity is lost, parasympathetic vagal activity continues unopposed. The response to hypoxia is bradycardia which can rapidly progress to asystole. Stimuli such as endotracheal intubation and tracheal suction can precipitate asystole.

Other treatment includes drainage of the stomach with a nasogastric tube and regular turning to avoid the development of pressure sores. Vasodilatation causes excessive heat loss. Every care should be taken to prevent hypothermia but not at the expense of being unable to examine or treat the patient adequately. The patient should not be allowed to become overheated as hyperpyrexia increases spinal cord oxygen consumption and may aggravate hypoxic damage due to other causes. High dose steroids have been claimed to reduce the degree of neurological deficit. Their value has not yet been proved conclusively but, if they are to be used, they should be given as soon as possible after the injury and certainly within eight hours. Methylprednisolone in a dose of 30 mg/kg/body weight has been recommended. This should be followed with an infusion given at 5.4 mg/kg/hour. The complications of high dose steroids, such as gastric ulceration, sodium retention, hyperglycaemia, delayed wound healing, increased risk of infection and anaphylactic shock must be carefully weighed against the potential benefits. Local hypothermia, diuretics, hyperbaric oxygen and calcium channel blockers have theoretical benefits but have not yet achieved general acceptance.

**Multiple injuries**.    Unless there is a high index of suspicion, a spinal cord injury may be missed in patients with multiple injuries. Conversely, the hypotension, respiratory embarrassment and loss of sensation due to the spinal cord injury may mask or confound the diagnosis of other injuries. The combination of a head and spinal cord injury is notorious for making other injuries difficult to diagnose. Management of the airway is the same, whatever the nature of the injuries. The adequacy of volume replacement can be extremely difficult to assess if there is both relative and absolute hypovolaemia. There is a tendency to err on the side of undertransfusion in order to reduce the risk of pulmonary oedema but, inevitably, this reduces tissue perfusion and may aggravate tissue hypoxia. Meticulous monitoring of fluid balance is essential and there is a good case for inserting a pulmonary artery flotation catheter in this type of patient.

**FURTHER READING**

Alderson, J.D. and Frost, E.A.M. (1990). *Spinal Cord Injuries: Anaesthetic and Associated Care*. London: Butterworths.

Gilbert, J. (1987). Critical care management of the patient with acute spinal cord injury. *Crit. Care Clin.*, **3**(3), 549–567.

# *Thoracic and lumbar spine injuries*

Thoracic and lumbar spine fractures without neurological deficit do not have specific implications for the anaesthetist although, as part of the team caring for the patient, the anaesthetist has a responsibility to ensure than his actions do not cause movement of the spine which may injure the spinal cord.

Injuries with an associated neurological deficit cause the same pathophysiological problems as cervical spine injuries but the changes become less as the level of the injury falls. Below T5, the problems are usually minimal and anaesthetic assistance at the time of admission is not required. Above T5, the patient requires individual assessment. There may be respiratory or cardiovascular abnormalities which require close monitoring in order to detect any deteriorations promptly.

# *Chest injury*

Rib fractures cause pain and inhibit adequate ventilation of the lungs and effective coughing. Provided that analgesia is provided, they usually heal without problems even if there is a flail segment present. Of far more importance to the anaesthetist is the underlying pulmonary contusion which can cause severe hypoxia and if inadequately treated is susceptible to infection and the development of the adult respiratory distress syndrome.

**Pathophysiology of pulmonary contusion**.  Pulmonary contusion consists of an area of parenchymal lung damage which heals by fibrosis surrounded by an area of atelectasis and oedema due to capillary damage. The area of atelectasis and oedema is amenable to treatment which, if effective, can dramatically alter the course of the recovery period. It has been clearly demonstrated that contused lung with minimal oedema and atelectasis recovers in 10 days and has a reduced, but sufficient, ability to resist infection. Contused and grossly oedematous lung takes far longer to recover and is totally unable to resist infection from inhaled bacteria. The oedema which develops in contused lung is increased by overtransfusion of any fluid but particularly by the overtransfusion of crystalloid solutions.

**Management of pulmonary contusion**.  Unless pulmonary contusion is severe, changes may not be apparent on chest X-ray until some hours after injury. Nevertheless, treatment is most effective if begun early. Oxygen should always be given.

Atelectasis is treated by providing adequate analgesia which enables the patient to cough, breathe deeply and cooperate fully with the physiotherapist. Intercostal nerve blocks, thoracic epidural analgesia or an intravenous infusion of opiate are all satisfactory methods of pain control. An opiate infusion may be contraindicated if the patient also has a head injury as is the use of intrathecal morphine which is another effective method of controlling pain. Local anaesthesia through an indwelling, intrapleural catheter is another method of pain relief.

The development of oedema is minimized by limiting the use of crystalloid solutions to 1 litre for resuscitation and to the minimum daily water requirement thereafter. The use of colloids and blood is not restricted. Indeed, it is vital that the circulating blood volume is restored to normal to ensure adequate tissue oxygenation. Overload with any type of fluid should be avoided. Central venous pressure monitoring is helpful and the use of a pulmonary artery flotation catheter is indicated if myocardial contusion or ischaemic heart disease complicate the pulmonary injury.

Antibiotics should be reserved until a chest infection has developed and the type of bacterium and its sensitivity is known. Steroids are effective in limiting the extent of oedema but increase the incidence of gram negative chest infections and, ultimately, are associated with a poorer outcome.

Mechanical ventilation is reserved for those patients whose respiratory function deteriorates in spite of the measures previously described and for those patients in whom there is combined head and chest injury when even minimal hypoxia may be deleterious to the brain.

There are still some centres where immediate mechanical ventilation is recommended for all patients with multiple rib fractures and those with a flail segment on the basis that internal pneumatic stabilization of the rib fractures will improve oxygenation and the eventual outcome. There are others particularly in Europe, who advocate internal fixation of rib fractures. The evidence that these methods of treatment are superior to any others is scanty. If, however, the patient needs a thoracotomy for treatment of injury to the heart, great vessels or oesophagus and the rib fractures are easily accessible, there is no doubt that fixation of the ribs will reduce post-operative pain and that a period of post-operative ventilation can be helpful.

**Other chest injuries**.  Fractures to the sternum, first rib and scapula rarely require specific treatment but should be viewed with suspicion as they indicate that the chest has received a severe blow and other, significant, thoracic injuries may be present. Diaphragmatic rupture is a relatively common injury which causes non-specific signs such as dullness at the base of the lung and decreased air entry into the lung. Bowel sounds heard in the chest can mean that bowel has herniated through the diaphragmatic rupture. This can be confirmed radiologically. Loops of bowel or the tip of a nasogastric tube may be seen within the chest. Other changes on the chest X-ray are less specific. They include an elevated hemidiaphragm or mediastinal shift. The management of severe haemorrhage due to myocardial rupture or tears in the major blood vessels, and massive air leaks from a ruptured trachea or bronchus, has already been described (p. 85). Oesophageal injury does not usually require treatment in the A&E department but prompt diagnosis is essential. Untreated, it can lead to fulminant mediastinitis. The diagnosis should be suspected if air is seen in the soft tissues of the neck or in the mediastinum and if a pleural effusion is smelly.

**Anaesthesia for chest injury**.   In the A&E department, this is rarely required except for life-saving procedures which have already been described (p. 83). It may become necessary at a later stage for the treatment of other injuries. This may influence the decision about whether a small pneumothorax should be drained in the A&E department. Because nitrous oxide is more soluble than nitrogen, its use will increase the size of an undrained pneumothorax. It is customary to drain all pneumothoraces before the induction of anaesthesia if a technique involving nitrous oxide is planned. Some anaesthetists would also place prophylactic chest drains in all patients with rib fractures who undergo anaesthesia with positive pressure ventilation even if a pneumothorax is not present and nitrous oxide will not be used. It should, however, be possible to detect the development of a pneumothorax during anaesthesia by close monitoring of arterial oxygenation which will decrease and inspiratory ventilatory pressures which will rise as the pneumothorax develops. There is merit in using local anaesthesia or avoiding anaesthesia altogether in patients with pulmonary contusion. This is because prolonged general anaesthesia is associated with atelectasis and depression of ciliary function, both of which increase the risk of chest infection.

**FURTHER READING**

Trinkle, J.K. and Richardson, J.D. (1981). Thoracic injuries. In *International Medical Reviews, Surgery* 1, *Trauma* (Carter, D.C. and Polk, H.C., eds). London: Butterworths, pp. 66–90.

# *Fractures of the long bones and pelvis*

These injuries, occurring in isolation, are unlikely to require an anaesthetist for their management unless angulation of the fracture is such that blood vessels are compressed and the viability of the limb is at risk. Anaesthesia may be requested but the fracture can often be reduced by a skilled surgeon using gentle traction, particularly if alcohol intoxication provides some analgesia.

Some fractures are associated with major blood loss and there is good evidence to show that inadequate resuscitation can cause the fat embolism syndrome which, in its severest form, causes gross hypoxia, pulmonary oedema, coma and sometimes death. The anaesthetist may therefore wish to assist with the resuscitation of patients with long bone or pelvic fractures in order to ensure that the fat embolism syndrome does not develop.

**The pathophysiology of fat embolism syndrome.** The fat embolism syndrome is characterized by widespread capillary endothelial damage. In the lungs, this causes hypoxia and interstitial oedema and in the brain petechiae cause a range of signs from mild confusion through to coma and brain stem death. The pathophysiological changes in the brain and lungs are the most usual causes of death but petechiae may also be found in the skin, retina and conjunctiva which may assist with diagnosis. Capillary damage is also detectable in the kidney, liver and other organs.

Most patients with long bone and pelvic fractures, who die shortly after injury, have fat globules in their lungs detectable at post mortem but do not necessarily show the clinical signs of the fat embolism syndrome prior to death. The mechanism which precipitates the development of fat embolism syndrome is not clearly understood. It is thought to be due to the breakdown of triglycerides into free fatty acids but the precipitating factors for this breakdown have not been elucidated. It is not clear whether these fatty acids then pass into the systemic circulation via the pulmonary circulation or whether fat globules pass into the systemic circulation via the foramen ovale and then breakdown into free fatty acids. The distribution of petechiae is immensely variable and does not correlate well with the severity of the syndrome. It is, for example, possible to have severe pulmonary fat embolism syndrome without the brain being affected and vice versa.

Numerous treatments have been suggested for preventing or reducing the pathophysiological changes of fat embolism syndrome but none have been conclusively shown to be useful. When the syndrome has developed, management is limited to supportive therapy. The incidence of fat embolism syndrome can, however, be reduced by prompt and effective immobilization of fractures in the A&E department.

**The prevention of fat embolism syndrome**.  Fat embolism syndrome does not usually develop for 24 to 48 hours after injury and is therefore not a diagnostic problem for the A&E doctor. There is some evidence that alcoholic intoxication is protective. The key to prevention is the administration of oxygen from the time of injury, rapid and effective volume resuscitation and the immobilization of fractures. The importance of the commencement of these measures in the A&E department cannot be overemphasized.

**FURTHER READING**

Cameron, P.D. (1990). Fat embolism. In *Intensive Care Manual* (Oh, T.E., ed.). Sydney: Butterworths, pp. 187–191.

# Pulmonary aspiration of blood and vomit

The inhalation of blood and vomit is, in theory, a preventable cause of morbidity and mortality in the injured patient. Total prevention is difficult to achieve because inhalation may occur in the unconscious patient before the emergency services arrive.

**Pulmonary inhalation of blood.** This occurs in unconscious, head injured patients who are bleeding from the base of the skull, the nose or the mouth. Inhalation of blood clots can cause obstruction of the trachea or large airways and distal collapse of the lung. Removal at bronchoscopy should be possible. More commonly, a steady trickle of blood is inhaled into the lungs and migrates to the periphery where it blocks the alveoli and prevents diffusion of oxygen across the alveolar membrane. Bronchoscopy and bronchial lavage are rarely helpful and treatment is supportive. Hypoxia can be extremely severe and controlled mechanical ventilation with 100% oxygen is sometimes necessary for two to three days. Fortunately, the lungs are efficient at scavenging blood which does not cause permanent pulmonary damage. If adequate oxygenation can be maintained until the blood begins to clear, the patient usually makes an uneventful recovery.

**Inhalation of gastric contents.** The pathophysiological picture depends on the nature of the inhaled gastric contents. Solid food causes similar problems to the inhalation of large clots of blood and the treatment is the same. The inhalation of liquid stomach contents may cause transient hypoxia and bronchospasm but very rarely significant lung damage. This is because it is unusual for most people to go more than four hours between meals and commonly accidents occur at shorter intervals than this after a meal. The stomach stops emptying at the time of the accident and the remaining food is sufficient to neutralize the acid which is secreted.

The inhalation of acidic stomach contents is rare in the seriously injured patient. If it does occur, it causes chemical damage to the alveolar capillary membrane. The patient becomes hypoxic due to interstitial oedema and is at greater risk of developing pulmonary oedema due to fluid overload. The first and most important measure is to ensure adequate oxygenation. Initially oxygen should be administered through a face mask. If inhalation occurred during endotracheal intubation, or if there is a risk of further vomiting and inhalation or if the patient is breathing inadequately as a result of the inhalation episode, endotracheal intubation to protect the airway and controlled mechanical ventilation are indicated. Some stomach contents may be retrieved by suction of the trachea and small solid particles may be more easily removed if suction is used in conjunction with saline lavage of the lungs. Liquid, acidic stomach contents pass rapidly to the peripheries of the lung. There is little evidence that lavage with an alkali such as sodium bicarbonate is helpful but there is evidence that alkaline solutions are capable of causing capillary endothelial damage. Hypovolaemia due to haemorrhage is aggravated by plasma leakage into the lungs and greater than normal volumes may be required for resuscitation. The patient may also develop acute bronchospasm which should be treated with a bronchodilator such as aminophylline and, if this fails, adrenaline. Reflex cardiac arrest can occur which is catastrophic if the patient is hypovolaemic secondary to haemorrhage from other injuries. Normal cardiac arrest procedures should be commenced in conjuncion with the rapid infusion of colloid and blood. Hydrocortisone may be helpful in the management of intractable bronchospasm but does not improve the overall outcome. Prolonged use of steroids increases the incidence of pulmonary infection by gram negative organisms and the ultimate mortality rate in the same way as when they are given to patients with pulmonary contusion. Antibiotics should not be given unless there is evidence of infection.

**Prevention of the pulmonary inhalation of blood and gastric contents**. In the A&E department the primary method of preventing pulmonary aspiration is protection of the compromised airway with an endotracheal tube. If the patient is deeply unconscious, the airway reflexes may be sufficiently obtunded for a tube to be passed without any form of anaesthesia. Often, anaesthesia and muscle relaxation are required. It is usually necessary to intubate the patient without delay. Emptying the stomach by passing a gastric tube or administering intravenous metoclopramide is inappropriate. In order for antacids such as magnesium trisilicate or sodium citrate to become effective in neutralizing stomach contents, time must be allowed for mixing. If the patient is unconscious, there will also be a delay while a nasogastic tube is passed for administration of the antacid. Such delays are rarely acceptable. The administration of $H_2$-receptor antagonists such as ranitidine or cimetidine serve only to stop the secretion of further acid and do nothing to reduce the risks of pulmonary acid aspiration during intubation in the A&E department. The prevention of pulmonary inhalation in the A&E department is limited to the use of cricoid pressure to prevent regurgitation of stomach contents and the judicious use of anaesthetic agents to minimize the risk of gagging and vomiting. The skill of the anaesthetist in rapidly securing the airway is also important as any delay in securing the airway increases the risk of aspiration.

# Mass casualties

# Problems caused by the admission of mass casualties

Major disasters have occurred throughout the history of the National Health Service. Most regions have a disaster plan which includes plans for the distribution of casualties to a number of local hospitals. In theory, therefore, each hospital should receive only the number of casualties with which it can easily cope. In the event of a major disaster, these plans do not always function as expected and the medical and nursing staff in the A&E department must be prepared to deal with large numbers of casualties in less than ideal conditions.

Each hospital also has its own disaster plan with which all staff should be familiar. The hospital plan will list the duties expected of each doctor. A few anaesthetists will be designated to work in the A&E department.

When faced with a number of severely injured casualties, the problem lies in knowing which to treat first so that the greatest number of lives can be saved. One doctor, usually a surgeon, will be designated to triage patients into categories as they pass through the front door of the hospital. Patients are usually divided into four groups:

1. Those requiring urgent resuscitation and/or surgery.
2. Those requiring resuscitation and/or surgery but who can wait for treatment.
3. Those with minor injuries who can wait until the more seriously injured have been treated.
4. Those who are dead or moribund and have no hope of survival, whether or not treatment is given.

During the first hours after a major disaster, the anaesthetist will probably be called upon to assist with the management of patients in the first group. Even after triage, there may be more patients than doctors available to treat them. In this situation it is common for each doctor to be given a group of patients to care for. This doctor may have to manage these patients without the assistance of other doctors and with a limited amount of help from nurses and other paramedics. In summary, the team approach to the care of the seriously injured, which is advocated elsewhere in this book, may not be a reasonable management option if a major disaster occurs.

It is essential, therefore, that every doctor has a prepared plan of action so that he can treat the greatest number of patients to the greatest benefit of each individual patient. In essence, the plan must include an approach to the management of several patients which encompasses a method of prioritizing the treatment of the life-threatening problems of major injury; namely, airway, breathing and circulatory insufficiency.

**FURTHER READING**

Haywood, I. (1988). Triage. *Care Crit. Ill.*, **4**, 12–14.

# *Assessing the severity of injury in mass casualties*

There are several scoring systems which can be used to assess the severity of injury. They are based on a physiological or anatomical assessment of the patient's problems. In general, the physiological scores are more appropriate for assessing the relative severity of injury in mass casualties. This is because, during the first phase of resuscitation, it is the physiological derangement of the respiratory and circulatory systems which causes life-threatening hypoxia and hypovolaemia. Use of a physiological scoring system not only allows the doctor to estimate the severity of the physiological derangement but also ensures that airway, breathing and circulation are assessed.

**Physiological scoring systems**.    There are two systems which are widely used. These are the Trauma Score (Table 1.5.1) and Revised Trauma Score (Table 1.5.2). These systems have been used for many years by paramedics in the United States and have been shown to correlate well with mortality. All patients with a Trauma Score of 13 or less are transferred to a Trauma Centre as are all patients with a coded score of less than four in any one of the three parameters used for measuring the Revised Trauma Score. In the mass casualty situation, the scores can be used to assess which patients have the greatest physiological derangement and as a guide to which patients require treatment most urgently. It must be emphasized, however, that the use of these scores is not an infallible guide to either injury severity or the need for urgent treatment. The validity of the scores has not been assessed in

**Table 1.5.1 The trauma score**

| | | |
|---|---|---|
| Respiratory rate | 10–24/min | 4 |
| | 25–35/min | 3 |
| | 36/min or greater | 2 |
| | 1–9/min | 1 |
| | 0/min | 0 |
| Respiratory expansion | Normal | 1 |
| | Retractive | 0 |
| Systolic blood pressure | 90 mmHg or greater | 4 |
| | 70–89 mmHg | 3 |
| | 50–69 mmHg | 2 |
| | 0–49 mmHg | 1 |
| | Impalpable pulse | 0 |
| Capillary refill | Normal | 2 |
| | Delayed | 1 |
| | None | 0 |
| Glasgow Coma Scale score | 14–15 | 5 |
| | 11–13 | 4 |
| | 8–10 | 3 |
| | 5–7 | 2 |
| | 3–4 | 1 |

**Table 1.5.2 The revised trauma score**

| Respiratory rate | Systolic blood pressure | Glasgow Coma Score | Score |
|---|---|---|---|
| 10–28 | 89 or greater | 13–15 | 4 |
| 29 or greater | 76–88 | 9–12 | 3 |
| 6–9 | 50–75 | 6–8 | 2 |
| 1–5 | 1–49 | 4–5 | 1 |
| 0 | 0 | 3 | 0 |

the very young or the very old. Furthermore, if the patient reaches hospital rapidly or is very fit and able to compensate effectively for blood loss, he may achieve a high score initially but deteriorate later if treatment is not begun promptly.

**Anatomical scoring systems**. The most widely used scores are the Abbreviated Injury Score and the Injury Severity Score. In the mass casualty situation, these scoring systems are unhelpful because they require a complete inventory of the injuries which will not be available until the secondary survey is complete.

**Combined physiological and anatomical scoring systems**. The CRAMS score (Table 1.5.3) has been used to assess injury severity and has been shown to correlate reasonably well with survival. It has some advantage over purely physiological scores because it includes an assessment of the abdomen which may be a source of occult and initially well compensated haemorrhage. Its disadvantage is that the range

**Table 1.5.3 The CRAMS score**

| | |
|---|---|
| Circulation | |
| Normal capillary refill or systolic BP greater than 100 mmHg | 2 |
| Delayed capillary refill or systolic BP 85–99 mmHg | 1 |
| Absent capillary refill or systolic BP less than 85 mmHg | 0 |
| | |
| Respiration | |
| Normal | 2 |
| Laboured, shallow or greater than 35/minute | 1 |
| Absent | 0 |
| | |
| Abdomen | |
| Abdomen and thorax not tender | 2 |
| Abdomen and/or thorax tender | 1 |
| Abdomen rigid, thorax flail or penetrating injury to either | 0 |
| | |
| Motor | |
| Normal, obeys commands | 2 |
| Responds only to pain, no posturing | 1 |
| Posturing or flaccid in response to pain | 0 |
| | |
| Speech | |
| Normal, orientated | 2 |
| Confused or inappropriate words | 1 |
| Unintelligible words or silence | 0 |

of possible scores is small and, therefore, it is not a good discriminator of injury severity.

The TRISS scoring system uses the Injury Severity Score and a weighted version of the Revised Trauma Score. It is not a suitable method for triage.

# Single-handed management of more than one patient

The physiological scoring systems described on p. 107 may provide some initial guidance as to which patients require treatment most urgently. The anaesthetist is still faced with planning the practicalities of the management of the patients in his care. To this end, attendance at an Advanced Trauma Life Support course can be helpful. These courses are designed to provide the doctor with a plan of management for a seriously injured patient which can be carried out by a doctor single-handed.

The anaesthetist may still be placed in a situation where there is more than one patient who, under normal circumstances, would be treated immediately. The reader may wish to give some thought to the situation in which he is asked to manage the following three patients:

*Patient 1.* This patient has a severe head injury, a fractured femur and fractured pelvis. He is unconscious, is unable to maintain his airway but with manual manipulation of the airway has a normal respiratory rate and pattern.

*Patient 2.* This patient is conscious and complaining of severe chest pain, is breathing shallowly and has no obvious respiratory excursion of the left side of the chest.

*Patient 3.* This patient is confused, is breathing rapidly and has thready peripheral pulses. There are obvious fractures of both femurs and the abdomen appears distended.

In summary, the first patient has a severe head injury with airway obstruction and potential hypovolaemia, the second has a chest injury with possible pneumothorax which could develop into a tension pneumothorax and the third has severe hypovolaemia due to bleeding from his fractures and a probable intra-abdominal injury.

Patients 1 and 3 obviously require immediate treatment and patient 2 could do so if a tension pneumothorax develops. Different doctors would probably treat these three patients in a variety of ways and it is possible to justify more than one approach.

Flexibility is the the key to success. Nevertheless, in a crisis, it is helpful to have a general plan of management. The simplest, quickest, effective treatment must be given to each patient. One approach is to treat patients with airway and breathing difficulties first. This is because hypoxia is life threatening and the patient cannot compensate as effectively for hypoxia as is possible for hypovolaemia. Furthermore, if circulatory compensatory mechanisms fail and the blood pressure falls, bleeding often ceases temporarily, only to start again as soon as resuscitation is commenced.

Using this approach patient 1 would be treated first to ensure an adequate airway. An oral airway might suffice but if there is any doubt an endotracheal tube would be used. A thoracostomy tube would then be inserted into the chest of patient 2 and with this in place self-administered Entonox could be offered for pain relief. Finally, one or more intravenous cannulae would be placed in patient 3 and rapid volume replacement commenced. Patient 1 could then be reassessed and if his breathing had become inadequate, controlled mechanical ventilation commenced if this had not already been done. An intravenous infusion might also be set up. Patient 2 would probably benefit from the insertion of an intravenous cannula and possibly some analgesia administered intravenously. By the time these actions are completed the initial volume replacement for patient 3 should be progressing well and a further assessment of his circulatory status could be made.

The reader may not agree with these suggestions and some would argue that as paitent 2 is conscious and has not yet developed a tension pneumothorax, it would be better to treat patient 3 before patient 2. The problem with the management of mass casualties is that there is never an ideal or correct solution to the problems which may arise. It is a valuable exercise for the anaesthetist to imagine a variety of mass casualty scenarios and to decide a plan of action for these patients. A leisurely bath is an ideal situation in which to ponder these problems.

# Life-threatening problems of burns

## *Hypoxia, hypovolaemia and myocardial failure*

Airway obstruction, difficulty with breathing and circulatory collapse threaten the lives of patients with severe burns just as they do the lives of patients with severe injuries. The number of potential causes for airway obstruction and breathing difficulty are fewer than for patients with non-burn injury. Cardiovascular collapse is nearly always due to plasma loss although rarely it may be due to myocardial depression by 'burn toxins' or poisonous gases. The management of burned patients is, therefore, more amenable to the use of protocols than the management of the non-burn patient and the use of a protocol is more likely to be appropriate for the individual patient's needs.

114

The approach to the acute management of a burn injury is the same as for patients with non-burn trauma; namely, a primary survey to identify airway, breathing and circulatory abnormalities, life-saving treatment to establish a clear airway, adequate ventilation of the lungs and to commence fluid replacement, a secondary survey to assess the precise extent and nature of the burn injury, definitive treatment and finally reassessment of the patient to identify discrepancies between the expected and actual effects of treatment. A significant proportion of burn injuries are due to house fires, explosions, electrocutions and automobile accidents. Patients burned in these type of accidents may also suffer non-burn injuries. These should be anticipated and specifically excluded during the secondary survey.

Although burn injury can be managed using protocols based on the anatomical assessment of the cutaneous injury, a pathophysiological approach to management is possible and, in certain circumstances, may result in more effective treatment. There are always individual variations in response to treatment. Furthermore, the magnitude of fluid loss is increased in patients with smoke inhalation and with electrical burns. In both cases, the extent of the cutaneous burn does not necessarily reflect the severity of the injury to subcutaneous tissues. Furthermore, the precise volume of fluid replacement required cannot be predicted accurately for these injuries. The pathophysiological approach to management is, therefore, mandatory.

## FURTHER READING

Martyn, J.A.J. (1990). *Acute Management of the Burned Patient*. Philadelphia: W. B. Saunders Co.

# The pathophysiological effects of burn injury

In the first few days after a burn injury, death is usually due to hypoxia, hypovolaemia or myocardial failure. Prompt resuscitation and treatment can save lives. Hypoxia may be due to upper airway swelling as a result of thermal injury, mechanical upper airway obstruction secondary to coma due to carbon monoxide or cyanide poisoning and pulmonary damage due to smoke inhalation. Hypovolaemia is due to leakage of plasma from burned tissue. Myocardial failure can be due to poisoning by carbon monoxide or cyanide and also from 'toxins' released from burned tissues. The causes of hypoxia, hypovolaemia and myocardial failure are specific to burn injury. Their pathophysiological effects, however, are identical to the pathophysiological effects of hypoxia, hypovolaemia and myocardial failure caused by non-thermal injury, namely, tissue hypoxia.

Tissue hypoxia, from whatever cause, leads to cellular dysfunction and cell death, the clinical manifestation of which is multiple organ failure. Multiple organ failure may develop in the burned patient if resuscitation has been suboptimal. It may also develop several weeks after the burn as a complication of sepsis.

In conclusion, multiple organ failure is a problem common to major trauma and burned patients. In both types of patient, an increase in mortality rate can be correlated to an increasing number of organ failures and to increasing severity and duration of hypoxia and hypovolaemia. In the burned patient, just as in the trauma patient, it is vital that hypoxia, hypovolaemia and myocardial failure are promptly recognized and effectively treated.

# *Reasons for failure of cellular oxygenation*

The discussion in this section refers specifically to changes associated with burn injury. It should be read in conjunction with the equivalent section on cellular oxygenation for non-burned patients (pp. 11–17) where the general principles of cellular oxygenation are described.

**Inhaled oxygen concentration**.   High inspired concentrations of oxygen are beneficial to all hypoxic and hypovolaemic patients. In the severely burned patient, these problems may be more severe than in the some injured patients particularly if the burn is associated with carbon monoxide or cyanide poisoning when the administration of 100% oxygen during life-saving resuscitation is mandatory. For some patients with severe carbon monoxide poisoning, hyperbaric oxygen will increase the speed of recovery and may reduce the incidence and severity of complications.

**Transfer of oxygen to the trachea and bronchial tree**.   There are two major causes of upper airway obstruction in the burned patient. The first is thermal injury to the larynx and glottis which results in swelling and narrowing of the airway. The second is loss of airway control due to a decrease in conscious level. This is usually due to severe carbon monoxide or cyanide poisoning but may be due to profound hypotension secondary to hypovolaemia.

Hypoxia may also occur due to poor respiratory excursion. Pain is rarely severe enough to limit respiratory excursion but painless, circumferential, full thickness burns of the chest wall may do so. Gas flow may be reduced due to narrowing of the bronchioles and lower airways by mucosal oedema. The trachea dissipates heat efficiently. Thermal burns of the lower airway are rare unless super-heated steam is inhaled. More commonly, oedema in the lower airways is secondary to chemical burns. Polyvinyl chloride, polyurethane, Teflon and Melamine are used widely in houses and release a variety of toxic products which include hydrogen chloride, phosgene, chlorine, formaldehyde, ammonia and hydrogen cyanide. Burning wood and paper produce acrolein which is also injurious to airways. In addition to causing chemical damage to the airways, these compounds are irritants and may provoke bronchospasm.

**Transfer of oxygen from the bronchial tree to the alveolar capillary membrane**. In the burned patient, the alveoli are usually well expanded unless a large airway has been obstructed by inhaled solid food or sloughing of the airway endothelium. The alveolar membrane may be obscured by carbon particles or pulmonary oedema secondary to chemical damage, myocardial failure or a combination of both. Massive alveolar disruption is uncommon unless the victim has been injured in an explosion.

**Transfer of oxygen across the alveolar capillary membrane to the blood**. The major limiting factor for transfer of oxygen across the alveolar capillary membrane in the patient with smoke inhalation is interstitial oedema secondary to the toxic contents of smoke.

Carbon monoxide has a binding affinity for haemoglobin which is at least 200 times that of oxygen. Even small amounts of carbon monoxide will significantly reduce the oxygen-carrying capacity of haemoglobin.

**Circulation of blood to the tissues**. In the first eight hours after a burn injury, there is a marked reduction in circulating plasma volume and hence cardiac output and blood flow to the tissues. Several mechanisms are involved. The most important are an increase in microvascular permeability in the area of burned tissue permitting plasma leakage, a generalized impairment of cell membrane function resulting in an increase in intracellular water and an increase in burn tissue osmotic pressure which leads to further accumulation of tissue fluid. Resuscitation commonly leads to intravascular hypoproteinaemia which is thought to be responsible for oedema formation in non-burned tissues. Oedema formation in non-burned tissues does not usually begin until six hours after burning but if there is a delay in admission to hospital and commencement of resuscitation, it can be an important contributor to hypovolaemia. The vasoconstrictor response is the same as for all types of hypovolaemia. As resuscitation commences and vasoconstriction is reversed, the patient becomes hypercatabolic and the circulation is hyperdynamic. These pathophysiological changes usually occur eight to 24 hours after burning and are not immediately relevant to the early resuscitation period. They should, however, be understood because resuscitation to parameters suitable for non-burn trauma and other hypovolaemic patients are ultimately insufficient for patients with large burns.

Myocardial failure in the early resuscitation phase is rare. It can, however, occur in patients with massive cutaneous burns when toxins which decrease myocardial contractility are released and in patients with carbon monoxide or cyanide poisoning severe enough to cause cellular hypoxia. Susceptible patients may suffer a myocardial infarction due to the stress of the injury or secondary to severe hypoxia or hypovolaemia.

**Transfer of oxygen from the capillaries to the tissues**. Patients with cutaneous burns of greater than 30% of the body surface area develop generalized capillary permeability and tissue oedema. This may increase the distance over which oxygen must diffuse from the capillaries to reach the tissues. Carbon monoxide shifts the oxygen dissociation curve to the left and decreases the amount of oxygen released to the tissues. Cyanide poisons the cytochrome oxidase enzyme system and inhibits intracellular energy production. Carbon monoxide is also thought to have a similar effect.

# *Treatment goals*

Hypoxia, hypovolaemia and myocardial failure are the three problems which pose a threat to life in burned patients. The treatment goals described for severely injured patients are equally applicable to burned patients. They are:

1. Ensure adequate oxygenation and ventilation of the respiratory tract.
2. Restore circulating blood volume to normal.
3. Optimize myocardial contractility.
4. Optimize arterial red cell content to facilitate oxygen transport and capillary blood flow.
5. Normalize erythrocyte oxygen affinity.

# Practical aspects

# *Ethical considerations*

It has been recognized for many years that there is a close association between age, area of cutaneous burn and mortality. In 1971 Bull published a mortality chart which clearly demonstrated this relationship. Since this chart was published, there have been many developments in the treatment of burns. Examples include improved management of hypovolaemia, early excision of burn wounds to reduce infection, new and powerful antibiotics and cardioactive drugs, recognition of the importance of adequate nutrition to aid healing and continuous arteriovenous haemofiltration for renal failure. These advances have improved the chance of survival but not as dramatically as might have been expected. This is perhaps because, as some traditional problems have been solved or ameliorated, the effect of smoke inhalation has become a significant contributor to mortality.

Cutaneous burns can cause gross disfigurement and physical disability. Again, advances in plastic and reconstructive surgery have reduced the distress that these can cause but often at the price of repeated hospital admissions and painful surgery.

In spite of these developments, there is a small group of patients who will not survive even when the best of current medical treatment is given. This group of patients includes all those aged 65 or more with cutaneous burns affecting more than 70% of the body surface area. For patients aged over 80, a burn affecting 60% of the body surface area is uniformly fatal. Sepsis is the usual cause of death. It is likely that during the lifetime of this book, the introduction of monoclonal antibodies and the use of cultured skin may alter the figures quoted.

Nevertheless, in the foreseeable future, there are always likely to be a few patients who will die whatever treatment they are given. Unlike predictors of mortality for other injuries and illnesses, the mortality chart of Bull, when used in conjunction with the data on probability of death from smoke inhalation, identifies a group of patients who lie in an area of the chart where death can be guaranteed. Other predictors of mortality are based on statistical calculations which are limited to identifying a mortality rate of 100% and do not indicate whether the patient is on the borderline between 100 and 110% mortality or well above the 100% mortality band.

Because the burns mortality chart is able to predict the ultimate death of some patients with absolute certainty, it is reasonable to question whether it is right to treat these patients in an aggressive manner in a futile attempt to save life or whether it is better to ensure that their comfort is guaranteed, that the process of dying is not prolonged excessively and that they are spared unnecessary and painful procedures. There are some who would argue that the patient and his relatives should be consulted at length and that this type of decision should not be made in the A&E

department. Furthermore, the procedures undertaken in the A&E department will probably be necessary, whatever the final decision. Intubation for airway obstruction, for example, will prevent the patient suffering the unpleasantness of choking for air. Similarly, adequate fluid replacement will prevent the sensation of thirst. There are others who would argue that prophylactic intubation, aggressive fluid management and the use of inotropic drugs are contraindicated in these patients.

Those working in the A&E department will be faced with these ethical dilemmas. The A&E doctor may not feel able to make such decisions without the advice of colleagues in the Burns Unit who probably have far more experience and are faced with coping with the results of decisions made by A&E doctors. It is better that the problem has been thought through and discussed with colleagues before the doctor finds himself in such a situation when decisions must be made in haste.

### FURTHER READING

Bull, J.P. (1971). Revised analysis of mortality due to burns. *Lancet*, **ii**, 1133–1134.

Clark, C.J., Reid, W.H., Gilmour, W.H. and Campbell, D. (1986). Mortality probability in victims of fire trauma: revised equation to include inhalational injury. *Br. Med. J.*, **292**, 1303–1305.

Hinds, C.J. (1992). Monoclonal antibodies in sepsis and septic shock. *Br. Med. J.*, **304**, 132–133.

# Estimating the extent and depth of cutaneous burns

The estimation of the extent and depth of a burn is of primary importance because fluid requirements can be reasonably accurately calculated if this information is available. It is also important because partial thickness burns are very painful and analgesia may be required. Full thickness burns to the face and neck can make intubation difficult and circumferential full thickness burns may restrict movement of the chest wall or circulation to the limbs.

**Surface area of cutaneous burns**.   The 'Rule of Nines' is a crude guide to the extent of the burned area and is useful during the primary survey. In adults the head and each arm are equal to 9% of the body surface area, the perineum is 1% and the anterior trunk, posterior trunk and leg are equivalent to 18% each. These figures are inaccurate for children in whom the head and legs are proportionately greater in area (Table 2.2.1). If the burn is patchy, the patient's closed palm and fingers are equal to an area of one per cent of his body surface area.

**Depth of cutaneous burn**.   Cutaneous burns may be divided into three types. Erythema consists of reddening of the most superficial layers of the epidermis. It is painful but does not blister and does not cause plasma loss. For the purposes of estimating burn wound size, erythema should be ignored.

In partial thickness burns, the epidermis and superficial layers of the dermis are destroyed. Nerve endings in the deeper layers of dermis are preserved so the wound is painful. Some epidermal cells which line the hair follicles

Table 2.2.1 Percentage body surface areas by age

|  | Neonate | 1y | 5y | 10y | 15y | Adult |
|---|---|---|---|---|---|---|
| Head | 19 | 17 | 13 | 11 | 9 | 7 |
| Neck | 2 | 2 | 2 | 2 | 2 | 2 |
| Upper limb | 9.5 | 9.5 | 9.5 | 9.5 | 9.5 | 9.5 |
| Front of trunk | 13 | 13 | 13 | 13 | 13 | 13 |
| Back of trunk | 13 | 13 | 13 | 13 | 13 | 13 |
| Buttocks and genitalia | 6 | 6 | 6 | 6 | 6 | 6 |
| One thigh | 5.5 | 6.5 | 8 | 8.5 | 9 | 9.5 |
| One leg | 5 | 5 | 5.5 | 6 | 6.5 | 7 |
| Foot | 3.5 | 3.5 | 3.5 | 3.5 | 3.5 | 3.5 |

deep in the dermis are preserved and a partial thickness burn will heal by repopulation from these epidermal sources. A partial thickness wound is soft to the touch and may be blistered or grossly swollen. Testing for sensation to pin prick is helpful in assessing burn depth. Partial thickness cutaneous burns do not ususally cause problems for the anaesthetist except when the larynx is involved because swelling may cause complete airway obstruction. Plasma loss occurs from partial thickness burns and may require replacement.

Full thickness burns are insensitive to pin prick and are leathery to the touch. The burn may extend in to subcutaneous tissues such as fat, muscle and even bone. Because the burn is rigid, oedema formation occurs but external swelling is restricted. The circulation to the limbs may be impaired as may chest wall excursion. Full thickness burns of the neck may cause massive swelling of the oropharynx and lead to airway obstruction. Furthermore, extension of the neck prior to intubation may be severely restricted. It may be impossible to feel the angle of the jaw or to use the jaw thrust manoeuvre to maintain the airway. Mouth opening may be restricted. Plasma loss from full thickness burns requires replacement.

# *The diagnosis of smoke inhalation, carbon monoxide and cyanide poisoning*

Any patient trapped in an enclosed space by a fire is likely to have inhaled smoke. Even those who have managed to escape may admit to inhaling smoke. It is usually impossible to know precisely what toxic substances the smoke contained. Various patterns of injury can occur.

**Smoke inhalation**.    All patients who have been trapped in a smoke-filled area or who give a history of inhaling smoke should be regarded as being at risk of pulmonary injury. Further clues that smoke inhalation has occurred include facial cutaneous burns, burns of the oropharnx, singed nasal vibrissae, soot in the mouth or expectoration of carbonaceous sputum. Smoke often contains carbon monoxide. A raised carboxyhaemoglobin level will identify patients at risk of developing pulmonary problems but not the severity of the problems. Initially the patient is unlikely to have difficulty breathing and the chest X-ray appears normal. Over the next few hours, laryngeal swelling may cause stridor of increasing severity and chemical injury to the lower airways may lead to bronchospasm which can become so severe that the patient requires controlled mechanical ventilation. Patients with smoke inhalation who are admitted to the A&E department shortly after injury rarely require treatment in the department. If the patient has inhaled smoke, he should be admitted for observation for 24 hours during which time significant laryngeal or pulmonary damage will become apparent. If a transfer by ambulance to a burns centre is being contemplated, consideration should be given to the possibility of breathing difficulties occurring during the journey and the advisability of prophylactic endotracheal intubation and ventilation. This should only be necessary if the journey will take more than an hour.

**Carbon monoxide poisoning**.   Carbon monoxide poisoning may be most accurately diagnosed by measuring the carboxyhaemoglobin level in the blood. The value obtained can be extrapolated to indicate the highest level which must have been present when the person was trapped in the fire. The cherry red colour of the mucous membranes which is a classical sign of carbon monoxide poisoning is not always easy to detect although it may be seen in the burn wound where erythrocytes containing carboxyhaemoglobin are fixed in burned tissue. The absence of cherry red colouring should not be regarded as conclusive evidence that carbon monoxide poisoning has not occurred. Other signs of carbon monoxide poisoning (Table 2.2.2) tend to be non-specific but may be used in conjunction with blood carboxyhaemoglobin levels to confirm the diagnosis.

**Table 2.2.2 The effects of acute carbon monoxide poisoning**

| Blood carboxyhaemoglobin | Effect |
| --- | --- |
| <10% | Asymptomatic |
| 10–20% | Headache, confusion and nausea |
| 20–40% | Irritability, dizziness, fatigue, dimming of vision and impaired judgement |
| 40–59% | Hallucinations, ataxia, convulsions and coma |
| >60% | Death |

**Cyanide poisoning**.   The diagnosis of cyanide poisoning can be difficult to make unless the patient is known to have been exposed to it. Blood cyanide levels of 0.2 mg/l are toxic and levels above 1 mg/l are fatal. Unfortunately, it takes several days for blood cyanide levels to be measured. The most reliable sign of cyanide poisoning is a persistent metabolic acidosis or persistently raised blood lactate levels, both of which are indicators of prolonged tissue hypoxia due to poisoning of the cytochrome system. It has been suggested that treatment for cyanide poisoning should be given if the carboxyhaemoglobin level is above 15% because, in burned patients, the two types of poisoning often occur together.

# The causes and diagnosis of upper airway obstruction

The causes of upper airway obstruction in burned patients are similar to those listed for the patient with severe trauma (Table 1.1.1, p. 13). Swelling of the larynx or oropharynx is a common cause of upper airway obstruction in the burned patient. It should be suspected if there is a possibility that flames or hot smoke have been inhaled. Solid vomitus or false teeth may also obstruct the airway. Airway reflexes may be depressed due to severe hypoxia secondary to carbon monoxide poisoning, cyanide poisoning, or severe upper or lower airway swelling. Severe hypovolaemia secondary to oedema formation in the burn wound and alcohol or drug abuse can also reduce the effectiveness of airway reflexes. Combined head and burn injury is relatively uncommon but should be considered if the type of accident is compatible with both of these injuries.

The diagnosis of upper airway obstruction is made in the same way as it is for patients with major trauma (pp. 20–21).

**Assess the verbal response to questioning**.   See p. 20.

**Look for injury to the upper airway or signs of abnormal affect**.   Facial burns, burns to the oropharynx, soot in the mouth, singed nasal vibrissae and expectoration of carbonaceous sputum are all signs that laryngeal burns may be present. Dribbling indicates inability to swallow saliva and is a sign of pharyngeal burns with swelling. Because the pharynx is in close proximity to the larynx this sign must be taken seriously even though signs of laryngeal swelling may not yet be apparent.

Upper airway swelling rarely causes hypoxia until the obstruction is almost complete. Lower airway burns, however, cause hypoxia at an early stage. Mild hypoxia may render the patient uncooperative, abusive or mildly confused. These abnormalities of behaviour may also indicate mild carbon monoxide or cyanide poisoning. Severe poisoning causes unconsciousness.

**Listen for abnormal respiratory sounds**.   All the sounds described on p. 20 may be present in the burned patient and be due either to loss of consciousness or to laryngeal and oropharyngeal swelling. It is particularly important for the same person to repeatedly assess the severity of stridor. As the swelling of the larynx increases the stridor becomes more marked. Increasing stridor is an indication for urgent endotracheal intubation to secure the airway. Prior to complete obstruction of the airway, airflow is reduced to such an extent that stridor diminishes. This sign is an indication for emergency intubation and may not be detected if different people assess the severity of stridor at different times.

**Feel for air on expiration**.   Its absence in the presence of respiratory effort is a sure sign of airway obstruction.

**Smell the expired air**.   Many burned patients are alcoholics. Alcohol on the breath may suggest this diagnosis.

**Look for cyanosis**.   Cyanosis should always be sought. It may be difficult to detect if it is obscured by soot around the mouth and on the extremities. Carbon monoxide poisoning reduces the amount of deoxyhaemoglobin in the circulation and hence cyanosis will not be visible until the patient is grossly hypoxic. Pulse oximetry can be used to detect hypoxia but is useless in the presence of carbon monoxide poisoning because oximeters cannot distinguish between oxyhaemoglobin and carboxyhaemoglobin. Both are measured and hence the oximeter will indicate that the blood is well saturated when, in fact, it is not.

**Look for the use of accessory muscles of respiration**.   This sign should be sought but may not be as apparent as in the patient with non-burn injury. It is most helpful to look for the use of accessory muscles in areas of the body which are not burnt.

# Pitfalls in the diagnosis of upper airway obstruction

All the pitfalls described for trauma patients (pp. 22–23) are relevant to burned patients particularly if there is a combination of burn and non-burn injuries. The most important pitfall is confusion between stridor due to upper airway swelling and expiratory wheeze due to bronchospasm or lower airway swelling.

**Stridor or bronchospasm**. In the burned patient, stridor and bronchospasm commonly occur together. This is because hot inhaled smoke causes thermal burns to the larynx and although heat is dissipated by the trachea, inhalation of smoke containing acidic substances causes chemical burns to the lower airways. Laryngeal swelling causes stridor which is mainly heard on inspiration, whereas lower airway swelling causes bronchospasm which is mainly heard on expiration. Both stridor and bronchospasm can, however, be associated with noises on inspiration and expiration. In the first few hours after burn injury, bronchospasm due to irritation from toxic gases is the commonest cause of expiratory wheeze. As time goes by, swelling of the larynx and/or lower airways progresses and stridor, worsening expiratory wheezing or a combination of both are noted. Anteroposterior and lateral X-rays of the cervical spine may show laryngeal swelling. The administration of bronchodilators may reduce the severity of the wheeze but does nothing for stridor. Flow volume studies are the most reliable method of distinguishing between upper and lower airway obstruction but cannot easily be performed in the A&E department. It is almost impossible to offer practical guidelines which will conclusively distinguish between upper and lower airway burn injury in the A&E department. If there is any doubt about the patency of the upper airway, endotracheal intubation is essential.

**Chest wall or pulmonary injury**. In the burned patient it is usually possible to distinguish between chest wall and pulmonary injury. Pain from partial thickness burns is rarely severe enough to impede chest wall expansion. Full thickness burns are relatively rigid. If the chest wall is circumferentially affected by full thickness burns, chest expansion will be severely limited unless escharotomies are performed. In the immediate post-burn period, use of the accessory muscles of respiration is nearly always due to limitation of chest wall movement. Laryngeal and lower airway swelling, in contrast, occurs within hours rather than minutes of burn injury.

# Methods of airway control

This section should be read in conjunction with the section on methods of airway control described for patients with major trauma (pp. 24–30). Many of the methods described are suitable for burned patients and the general comments made in the preceding section apply. In this section, comments will be restricted to the special problems created by the presence of upper airway and facial cutaneous burns. All the methods are associated with problems in this type of patient. In general, it is safest to secure the airway as soon as possible after signs of laryngeal injury have become apparent. Patients without upper airway or cutaneous facial burns who are unconscious because of carbon monoxide poisoning or gross hypovolaemia may be managed in exactly the same way as previously described for head injured and other unconscious patients (pp. 86–91).

**Manual methods of airway control.** This method of airway management is unsuitable for burned patients with upper airway swelling as it does not circumvent the laryngeal swelling.

If the patient is unconscious and has cutaneous facial and neck burns but a patent larynx, the anaesthetist may attempt to control the airway manually for a short time. This can be extremely difficult to do because full thickness burns render the angle of the jaw impalpable and prevent extension of the neck. Releasing escharotomies of the neck may, if extensive, be helpful but cannot be relied upon to solve the anaesthetist's problems.

**Oesophageal obturator airway.** This method is unsuitable for patients with laryngeal swelling because it does not relieve the obstruction.

131

**Laryngeal mask.** The laryngeal mask does not relieve obstruction due to swelling but may be used as an aid to endotracheal intubation (pp. 26–27).

**Oral endotracheal intubation.** This is the method which many anaesthetists prefer. It may be difficult in the presence of full thickness burns to the face or neck for the reasons already described. Furthermore, mouth opening may be severely restricted by circumoral full thickness burns. If the patient is conscious anaesthesia may be required. Topical local anaesthesia is often impossible because copious salivation dilutes the anaesthetic. General anaesthesia may be required. An inhalational technique is preferable until the anaesthetist has established that an airway can be maintained using manual methods. Muscle relaxants may then be used.

Suxamethonium is contraindicated in burned patients from two days to two months after injury because it is associated with release of potassium from the burnt tissue and cardiac arrest. The evidence which led to the delineation of these time limits is sparse. There is at least one report of cardiac arrest following suxamethonium given within 24 hours of injury but it is not entirely clear whether the suxamethonium was the cause of the arrest. There are also animal experiments which suggest that muscle and synaptic membranes are abnormal for far longer than two months following burn injury. In the burned patient, it is probably best to avoid suxamethonium at all times unless there are compelling reasons for using it. Intubation is possible under deep inhalational anaesthesia or following the administration of atracurium or vecuronium. The risks of pulmonary inhalation of gastric contents using these latter methods must be balanced against the relatively small risk of cardiac arrest after giving suxamethonium.

When the endotracheal tube has been positioned in the trachea, it must be secured firmly with ribbon gauze. Sticky tape should not be used on burned tissue. Whatever method is used for securing the tube, its fixation should be checked regularly. The tape may become excessively tight as the face swells or loose as the swelling subsides.

**Nasotracheal intubation**.   Nasotracheal intubation is a suitable technique for use in burned patients unless there is gross burn injury to the nose. Local or general anaesthesia may be used with the provisos mentioned above.

**Cricothyroidotomy and tracheostomy**.   Both these techniques have a place in the acute management of the compromised upper airway in the burned patient. It is undesirable to place any type of semi-permanent tube through burned tissue in the neck because the burn wound inevitably becomes infected. As a life-saving measure a cricothroidotomy or tracheostomy should always be considered although there may be technical problems with their insertion through burned tissues because landmarks are difficult to palpate through full thickness burn.

# Additional factors affecting the management of upper airway obstruction

Normal anatomical variants and the risk of vomiting and regurgitation are important factors which may complicate airway control in the burned patient. Contrary to the expectations of inexperienced doctors, swelling of the lips secondary to cutaneous burns is rarely a problem although the patient's appearance may be alarming.

**The risk of vomiting and regurgitation**.   Unlike patient's suffering non-burn trauma, patients who are burned, and have airway problems, are less likely to have eaten within six hours of burning and therefore they are less likely to have retained stomach contents. Burn injury can, and does, occur at all times of day and night but those patients who are trapped in a burning room are more likely to have been asleep in bed when the fire started. Commonly, this type of patient is admitted in the early hours of the morning and has not eaten since the previous evening. Nevertheless, burn injury, like other injuries, can cause delay or cessation of stomach emptying. All patients should be regarded as being at risk of pulmonary aspiration of acidic stomach contents, particularly if endotracheal intubation is not indicated until several hours after the injury occurred.

Doctors working in the A&E department should, however, be wary of the patient who has been rescued from a smouldering bed. This type of patient has commonly fallen asleep while smoking a cigarette and is often intoxicated with alcohol. Alcohol may delay stomach emptying.

# The causes and diagnosis of respiratory insufficiency

The basic pathophysiological causes of respiratory insufficiency in the burned patient, namely upper airway obstruction, inadequate chest wall excursion, inadequate lung expansion, inadequate respiratory drive and inadequate gas exchange, are identical to those of patients with non-burn trauma. In the burned patient, however, there are specific causes which relate to the nature of the injury. These are summarized in Table 2.2.3 and discussed in the following sections.

As has already been stressed in previous sections, the burned patient may also have non-burn injuries and this possibility should always be considered when the patient is examined.

**Inadequate movement of the chest wall**. Circumferential, full thickness burns of the chest wall can severely restrict expansion. In order to make the diagnosis, it is vital that the

**Table 2.2.3 Causes of respiratory insufficiency in burned patients**

| | |
|---|---|
| 1. Upper airway obstruction | Laryngeal swelling |
| | Carbon monoxide poisoning |
| | Cyanide poisoning |
| | Alcohol or drugs |
| | Hypoxia |
| | Hypovolaemia |
| | |
| 2. Inadequate excursion of the chest wall | Circumferential full thickness burn |
| | Tight bandages |
| | |
| 3. Inadequate lung expansion | Inadequate chest wall excursion |
| | Bronchospasm |
| | Pneumothorax |
| | Haemothorax |
| | |
| 4. Abnormal respiratory drive | Carbon monoxide poisoning |
| | Cyanide poisoning |
| | Alcohol or drugs |
| | Hypoxia |
| | Hypovolaemia |
| | |
| 5. Impaired gas exchange | Pulmonary collapse |
| |   Soot |
| |   Pneumothorax |
| |   Endothelial sloughing |
| | Pulmonary oedema |
| | Inhaled blood or stomach contents |
| | Pulmonary contusion |
| | Inadequate pulmonary perfusion |
| |   Hypovolaemia |
| |   Myocardial failure |
| | |
| 6. Non-burn injury | Tables 1.1.1 and 1.2.1 (pp. 13 and 36) |

chest is carefully examined both front and back and that the depth of burn is accurately assessed.

The management of cutaneous burns varies from centre to centre. In some centres, the burn is covered with a dressing such as flamazine, gauze, cotton wool and crepe bandages. If the bandages are applied by inexperienced doctors or nurses, they may be wound around the chest or abdomen too tightly and cause restriction of chest wall or diaphragmatic movement. It should be easy to insert the flattened fingers of one hand between the crepe bandage and the cotton wool. If this is not possible, it is likely that the bandage is too tight.

**Inadequate lung expansion**. The commonest causes are inadequate excursion of the chest wall or diaphragm or bronchospasm due to irritant gases or mucosal swelling due to chemical burns to the lower airway. The history of the injury accompanied by careful examination of the chest wall and auscultation for expiratory wheeze will enable the correct diagnosis to be made.

Patients injured in an explosion may develop a pneumothorax or haemothorax. The diagnosis of these injuries has been described on p. 35.

**Abnormal respiratory drive**. In the burned patient, this is almost always due to hypoxia secondary to pulmonary injury, carbon monoxide or cyanide poisoning or gross hypovolaemia. The diagnosis is made by noting the history of the injury, particularly if cyanide poisoning is suspected, measuring arterial blood gases and carboxyhaemoglobin, and assessing the adequacy of the circulation.

In the presence of severe carbon monoxide or cyanide poisoning, hypoxia is severe and cerebral oedema may contribute to the inefficiency of respiratory drive. Urgent treatment is indicated before the diagnosis can be confirmed by CT scanning or intracranial pressure monitoring.

**Impaired gas exchange**. Gas exchange may be impaired by the presence of large amounts of soot in the airways and alveoli, by pulmonary oedema due to chemical damage or by blast injury to the lungs which causes pathophysiological changes identical to pulmonary contusion, namely alveolar disruption, haemorrhage, atelectasis and interstitial oedema. The chest X-ray may be relatively normal. The diagnosis is made by noting the history and observing the pulmonary secretions for soot, oedema and blood.

As with non-burn injury, inadequate pulmonary blood flow due to hypovolaemia will cause severe tissue hypoxia.

# General management principles for respiratory insufficiency and potential difficulties

For burned patients, the management of respiratory insufficiency depends on the recognition of pathophysiological changes and is, in principle, no different to the management of other patients with respiratory insufficiency. The administration of pure oxygen while other measures are instituted, provision of analgesia, restoration of circulating blood volume and commencement of mechanical ventilation are all indicated for the same reasons as discussed on pp. 39 and 40. Some measures are specifically appropriate to burned patients and routine measures may be complicated by cutaneous burns.

**Improving expansion of the chest wall**. If chest wall expansion is limited by circumferential, full thickness cutaneous burns, the solution is to perform extensive escharotomies. The relieving excisions must extend down to non-burned, vascular tissue. This tissue will be observed to bulge outwards as the incisions are made and the burned tissue edges of the escharotomy wound will separate by a centimetre or more. General anaesthesia is sometimes requested for escharotomies. When performed by a skilled surgeon, this procedure is almost painless because the cutaneous nerve endings have been destroyed and fat contains little nervous tissue. In general, the request for anaesthesia should be resisted unless the patient is obviously distressed. Sometimes, however, there is significant bleeding from blood vessels in the underlying viable tissue and these vessels require cauterization with a diathermy. This can be painful. In this situation, ketamine is a useful agent. It must always be given with midazolam to prevent hallucinations in the recovery period and there must always be facilities for endotracheal intubation and monitoring, although in the majority of cases the airway is well maintained.

137

If chest or abdominal bandages have been applied too tightly, they must be removed and applied more loosely.

**Drainage of the pleural cavity**. Cutaneous burns may be present in the sites normally advocated for drainage of air or blood in the pleural cavity. Because cutaneous burns frequently become infected, it may be necessary to place chest drains in sites which would normally be considered inappropriate. Effective drainage of the pleural cavity is facilitated if the drains are carefully directed within the cavity towards, or preferably into, their normal position. In life-threatening situations, the doctor should not hesitate to place a chest drain through burned tissue. The tube can, if necessary, be repositioned at a later stage.

**Inability to ventilate the lungs or achieve adequate oxygenation**. In the A&E department, these problems are rarely, if ever, related to the burn injury. The cause is usually due to equipment failure (p. 41). Severe bronchospasm occasionally causes extreme difficulty in achieving adequate ventilation. Management options are discussed on pp. 203–206.

# The causes and diagnosis of cardiovascular insufficiency

There are four major causes of cardiovascular collapse in the burned patient. These are summarized in Table 2.2.4.

**Major plasma loss**. Plasma loss, like blood loss, causes cardiovascular collapse due to hypovolaemia and is poorly tolerated by the old and infirm and well tolerated by athletes. A rise in pulse rate, fall in blood pressure and pulse pressure, and peripheral vasoconstriction should be sought but may be difficult to detect because of the difficulties of monitoring patients with cutaneous burns (pp. 143–148). The assessment

**Table 2.2.4 Causes of cardiovascular insufficiency in burned patients**

1. Cardiac arrest
   Severe hypoxia
   Severe hypovolaemia
   Myocardial failure due to burn 'toxins' or carbon monoxide/cyanide
     poisoning
   Dysrhythmias secondary to electrical shock

2. Tension pneumothorax

3. Massive unreplaced plasma loss

4. Non-burn injury
   Table 1.2.2 (p. 43)

of other parameters affected by hypovolaemia such as respiratory rate, urine output and mental status may therefore be vitally important, although it is important to distinguish between respiratory causes for an increase in respiratory rate, to note the presence of myoglobinuria which may be associated with impaired renal function (p. 145), and to be aware of hypoxia, alcohol intoxication, carbon monoxide poisoning and cyanide poisoning as possible causes of impaired mental function.

**Cardiac arrest**. In the burned patient, cardiac arrest is rarely due solely to hypovolaemia, although the presence of an inadequate circulating blood volume may hinder attempts to resuscitate the patient. Cardiac arrest is normally due to gross hypoxia secondary to carbon monoxide or cyanide poisoning and may be complicated by the specific myocardial depressant effects of these poisons. The diagnosis of these problems is described elsewhere (pp. 160 and 162).

Cardiac dysrhythmias may occur in patients who suffer a myocardial infarction prior to, or as a result of, the burn injury and in patients subjected to a high voltage electrical shock. Electrocardiographic monitoring is essential but may be hampered by cutaneous burns (pp. 146–147).

Cardiac arrest rarely occurs in patients with extensive cutaneous burns due to 'burns toxins' which have a depressant action on the myocardium. These toxins are probably similar to those released from hypoxic cells in non-burn trauma but are released in greater quantities and therefore have a more dramatic effect.

**Tension pneumothorax**. Tension pneumothorax should be suspected in all patients who have been burned in an explosion or who have been in an accident which may have caused other injuries. The diagnosis is discussed on pp. 45–47.

**Non-burn injury**. The causes of cardiac arrest due to non-burn injury are summarized in Table 1.2.2. (p. 43) and discussed on pp. 44–45.

# General management principles for cardiovascular insufficiency

The management of cardiovascular collapse depends on the diagnosis. As with severely injured patients, one or more large bore cannulae must be inserted as quickly as possible. The siting of the cannulae will depend mainly on the location of cutaneous burns. In a life-threatening emergency it is acceptable to cannulate a vein through burned tissue. If time is available it is preferable to place cannulae through unburned skin. Not only does this reduce the risk of infection, but also makes it far easier to secure the cannula in position. If a cannula is placed through burned tissue, suturing may be the only effective means of fixation. The A&E doctor may find that it is necessary to cannulate veins which would normally be avoided because of the risk of infection and the immobility which cannulation causes. Such veins include the femoral vessels and veins in the lower leg and feet. Severely burned patients are usually bedridden during the early stages of illness and the risk of deep vein thrombosis is reduced by anticoagulation. The risk of infection from a cannula in the femoral vein is often less than the risk from a cannula sited in burned tissue. In any event, cannulae used for resuscitation can be resited once resuscitation is well underway.

**Hypovolaemia.** All patients should be given oxygen. Fluid replacement should be commenced as quickly as possible. Various regimes are available (Table 2.3.1, p. 151) and most hospitals have a protocol. It is important to remember that these protocols are designed to administer an hourly volume of fluid calculated as if resuscitation commences immediately after injury. If there has been a delay between injury and the commencement of resuscitation, the volume of fluid given in the first hour must include not only that hour's calculated requirement, but also the volume for the hours which have passed since the injury occurred.

**Myocardial failure.** In the burned patient, myocardial failure results from gross hypoxia secondary to carbon monoxide or cyanide poisoning and from depression of activity by burns toxins. Failure from both causes is resistant to treatment. Myocardial failure is treated as described on pp. 199–201 although larger than normal doses of drugs may be required. In addition to the inherent resistance of the myocardium to inotropic drugs, burned patients also have altered drug metabolism. This alteration has multiple causes including alterations in circulating blood volume, loss of drugs in plasma escaping from burned tissue, altered protein binding, impaired hepatic and renal function and alterations in motor end plate function. Most of these changes have little significance in the A&E department and become relevant when long-term therapy is contemplated. Nevertheless, the A&E doctor should be aware of them as resuscitative measures may influence later management.

**Cardiac arrest.** Cardiac arrest is treated as described on pp. 182–185. The usual causes of cardiac arrest in the burned patient are hypoxia, hypovolaemia and myocardial failure.

Prompt correction of hypoxia due to airway or breathing abnormalities and the rapid infusion of fluid are essential if resuscitation is to be successful.

Electrocution can cause cardiac arrest from dysrhythmias. As long as gross myocardial muscle damage has not occurred, restoration of a normal rhythm may be achieved by standard methods (pp. 192–194). Myocardial damage due to electrocution produces a clinical picture similar to that of myocardial infarction and hence is treated in a similar manner. If cardiac arrest has occurred secondary to carbon monoxide poisoning, cyanide poisoning, or as a result of burn toxin myocardial depression, successful resuscitation is extremely unlikely.

**Tension pneumothorax**. The treatment is described on p. 49.

# Difficulties in the management of cardiovascular insufficiency

The three difficulties described for the severely injured patient, namely inability to secure venous access, inability to secure an improvement in the patient's condition and failure to make the correct diagnosis, are also encountered in burned patients.

**Inability to secure venous access**. The problems caused by cutaneous burns have already been described. The solutions are the same as described for severely injured patients (pp. 51–53).

**Failure to gain an adequate response to treatment**. If venous access is adequate, it most unlikely that it will be impossible to keep up with fluid losses. If the response is inadequate, it is probable that either the diagnosis has been incorrectly made or the calculation of fluid requirements is arithmetically incorrect. Whichever protocol is used, it should never be forgotten that strict adherence to a protocol is not always appropriate for every patient. The protocol is designed so that most patients will be treated adequately most of the time. Some patients will require less than the volume stated by the protocol and others will require more. Patients who routinely require more fluid include those with inhalational injury where interstitial and overt pulmonary oedema are responsible for significant volumes of plasma loss; those with electrical burns where the area of cutaneous burn is often small compared to the extensive subcutaneous and muscle damage which occurs secondary to coagulation of blood vessels, and those who have non-burn injuries which normally cause blood loss. Furthermore, myocardial failure may cause tachycardia and hypotension in a normovolaemic patient.

It is unwise to rely totally on a protocol. A pathophysiological approach to resuscitation which includes monitoring and interpretation of changes in physiological parameters is essential.

**Failure to make the correct diagnosis**.   Reassessment of the patient is essential when life-saving measures are well underway. In particular, the area of the cutaneous burn should be reassessed and the chest re-examined for signs of pulmonary complications which may not have been apparent or even suspected at the time of admission. Bronchospasm, radiological changes and deteriorating blood gases often become more apparent in the first few hours after admission. The presence of non-burn injuries should be sought.

# *Monitoring resuscitation and definitive treatment*

During life-saving resuscitation, the monitoring methods used will probably be relatively non-invasive. The general principles are the same as those employed for seriously injured patients but may be complicated or confounded by the presence of the burn injury. As with the seriously injured patient, it is desirable to monitor as many parameters as possible in order to facilitate the correct interpretation of abnormal findings. The methods described on pp. 54–63 are applicable to burns patients and the interpretations may be the same. In the following sections, special problems created by the burn injury are discussed.

**Eyes, nose, ears and hands**.　Look at the patient and assess all the features which may indicate airway or breathing difficulties. Look also for the features of hypovolaemia. Cutaneous burns and soot on normal skin may conceal some of the signs but it should be possible to glean enough information to make a correct diagnosis.

Smell the patient. Alcohol may be detected with the same implications as for the trauma patient. In addition, solvents or petrol may be detected. The burn may have been self inflicted or an act of aggression by another party.

Feel for air on expiration and for the temperature of the limbs. Cool peripheries could be a sign of hypovolaemia but may also indicate reduced blood flow to one limb as a result of tissue swelling within a circumferential full thickness burn. Palpation of the position of the trachea may not be possible due to full thickness burns but the presence of the burn may remind the anaesthetist that endotracheal intubation will be potentially difficult.

**Pulse oximetry**.　Pulse oximetry is a useful method of measuring arterial oxygen saturation. In addition to producing abnormal results in the presence of vasoconstriction, the reading will also be reduced if local limb blood flow is reduced. Most pulse oximeters are unable to distinguish between oxyhaemoglobin, carboxyhaemoglobin and methaemoglobin. In the presence of smoke inhalation and carbon monoxide poisoning, pulse oximetry may give a false sense of security.

**Non-invasive pulse and blood pressure**. Cutaneous burns often occur on the upper arms and make the placement of a cuff difficult but not necessarily impossible. The burn can be covered with Vaseline-impregnated gauze and a thin layer of dressing gauze topped by an occlusive plastic dressing such as Opsite® or Cling Film®. If the dressings are applied sparingly a cuff can be placed over the dressing and will enable the blood pressure and pulse rate to be measured without difficulty. If the dressing is found to be too bulky, a sterile cuff can be placed over a layer of Vaseline gauze. Alternatively, the cuff can be placed around an unburned ankle. Allowance must then be made for inaccuracies of measurement due to discrepancies in the size of the cuff compared to the circumference of the ankle. Even though the measurements obtained at the ankle may not be accurate when compared to blood pressure measured invasively, they are rarely so inaccurate as to be clinically unhelpful. It is still possible to detect trends in blood pressure and to monitor the progress of resuscitative measures.

**Capillary filling, venous filling and skin-core temperature difference**. These monitoring parameters are useful for detecting hypovolaemia although they may also be abnormal if there is a localized reduction in tissue blood flow.

**Urine output**. Measurement of urine output in the burned patient is a valuable guide to the adequacy of vascular filling. Severe burn injury is associated with the release of large quantities of antidiuretic hormone. Small volumes of highly concentrated urine are produced. During resuscitation the minimum acceptable urine output is 0.5 ml/kg body weight/hour and it is desirable to achieve an hourly volume of 1 ml/kg. Acute renal failure may occur very early in burned patients but is unlikely to concern doctors working in the A&E department. Trends in urine volume and concentrating power can be valuable in detecting the onset of renal impairment. For this reason, it is valuable to measure urine osmolarity in the A&E department. In the presence of electrical burns, flame burns which have involved muscle or extensive cutaneous burns, pigment may be noted in the urine. The pigment may be haemoglobin or myoglobin. In either case the patient is at risk of renal failure if adequate urine flow is not maintained. It is customary to increase urine flow with an osmotic diuretic such as mannitol. Sequential hourly measurements of urine volume do not then reflect the adequacy of fluid replacement although serial samples of urine will display a return to normal colouration and the reduction in risk from renal failure due to pigment.

**Level of consciousness**.   Although originally described as a monitoring tool for the assessment of head injuries, the Glasgow Coma Scale is helpful for describing all types of unconsciousness including that resulting from carbon monoxide poisoning. Carbon monoxide poisoning is commonly associated with the development of cerebral oedema secondary to hypoxia. Hence, monitoring the level of consciousness in patients known to have suffered severe carbon monoxide poisoning is valuable.

**Central venous pressure**.   Used correctly, the measurement of central venous pressure is helpful for monitoring the progress of fluid resuscitation. In the burned patient there may be practical difficulties in finding a suitable site for inserting the catheter. Immediately following burning, the wounds are sterile. It is therefore acceptable to insert a central venous catheter through burned tissue provided that it is removed after life-saving resuscitation is complete. Alternatively, the catheter may be inserted through burned tissue and then tunnelled so that it exits through unburned skin.

**Electrocardiogram**.   Monitoring of the electrocardiogram is essential if the patient has been electrocuted or has carbon monoxide or cyanide poisoning. It can also be a helpful monitor of heart rate while a site is located for the measurement of pulse and blood pressure. The location of cutaneous burns often makes it impossible to fix self-adhesive electrodes in standard positions. It is usually possible to find sufficient unburned skin to place electrodes in some form of triangle around the heart. This will enable rate and rhythm to be monitored although ischaemic changes are not reliably demonstrated. An alternative is to use needle electrodes inserted through the burned tissue. These are generally less effective as they have a tendency to fall out.

**Blood gas and end tidal carbon dioxide measurement**. If oxygen has been given and fluid resuscitation is adequate, the results obtained should be normal. A metabolic acidosis implies severe tissue hypoxia due to either persistent hypovolaemia or carbon monoxide or cyanide poisoning. During the recovery phase, burned patients become hypercatabolic and produce large volumes of carbon dioxide but this is not a problem during life-saving resuscitation.

**Full blood count**. In the burned patient, measurement of haemoglobin and haematocrit on admission may act as a useful guide to the adequacy of resuscitation. Plasma loss results in haemoconcentration. In the absence of other injuries or a pre-existing abnormality of haemoglobin concentration, the haematocrit can be used as a guide to the adequacy of resuscitation. As a general rule, fluid should be administered to maintain the haematocrit at around 40%. In the presence of active bleeding or pre-existing anaemia the absolute values should be interpreted with caution but trends are still useful. In the A&E department, erythrocyte loss in the burn wound and from escharotomies rarely causes significant anaemia but a transfusion of red cells is often necessary in the second 24 hours after injury. For regular monitoring capillary samples are sufficient, but at the time of admission venous blood must be taken for crossmatch and the blood count can be estimated from blood sampled at the same time.

**Urea, blood sugar and electrolyte estimation**. These serve as a useful baseline measurement as levels may alter during the first few days after burning.

147

**Carboxyhaemoglobin and cyanide estimations**. Regular measurement of carboxyhaemoglobin is helpful during resuscitation as the level correlates with the level of consciousness. Prolonged unconsciousness which does not correlate with blood carboxyhaemoglobin levels indicates either hypoxic brain damage, the development of cerebral oedema or that the unconsciousness is due to another cause such as concomitant head injury or severe alcoholic intoxication.

The measurement of cyanide levels is not immediately helpful because the results are not usually received for several days. The results can, however, be useful retrospectively as they may confirm that treatment administered immediately was indeed necessary, and may also explain untoward developments that might otherwise be of doubtful causation.

**FURTHER READING**

Barrett, M. (1986). Renal function following thermal injury. *Care Crit. Ill.*, **2**, 197–201.

# Definitive management

# *The definitive diagnosis of injuries*

As with serious non-burn injuries, it is usually possible to manage life-threatening burns by assessing and correcting pathophysiological abnormalities. Definitive management, however, is easier if an anatomical diagnosis of injuries is made.

**Surface area of cutaneous burns**.   The 'Rule of Nines' is a crude guide to the extent of the burned area and is useful during the primary survey. During the secondary survey a more accurate estimation of the area of cutaneous burn can be made using the figures given in Table 2.2.1, (p. 124).

**Depth of cutaneous burn**. The depth of the cutaneous burn will already have been assessed rapidly during the primary survey. The assessment should be repeated at leisure during the secondary survey. The assessment is likely to be more accurate and will, therefore, provide a better basis for calculating fluid requirements.

**Smoke inhalation**. All patients who have been trapped in a smoke-filled area or who give a history of inhaling smoke should be regarded as being at risk of pulmonary injury. The probability that smoke has been inhaled will already have been noted during the primary survey. By the time the secondary survey is made, upper and lower airway swelling will have increased and the signs of smoke inhalation may be more obvious. If pulmonary damage is severe, fluffy opacities caused by interstitial oedema may already be apparent on the chest X-ray although, with less severe injuries, X-ray abnormalities may not be seen until some hours after the injury.

**Carbon monoxide poisoning and cyanide poisoning**. See pp. 160 and 162.

# *Estimating fluid requirements*

Plasma loss from cutaneous burns has a relatively constant relationship to the surface area of the burn and the weight of the patient. As a general rule adults with cutaneous burns of greater than 15% of their body surface area and children with burns of greater than 10% require intravenous replacement fluids. They are traditionally referred to as 'shock cases'. Numerous regimes are available for estimating the volume of replacement fluid required. Examples are shown in Table 2.3.1 (p. 152). It should be noted that the volume of fluid suggested by a particular regime does not necessarily correlate with the volume of plasma lost because the replace-

fluid is not always identical in content and osmolarity to plasma. Perusal of the many regimes available indicates that an average figure for plasma loss in the first 24 hours after injury is 2 ml/% area burn/kg body weight.

The rate of plasma loss is maximal in the first eight hours after injury and gradually declines over the next 40 hours. This is because in burned tissues large endothelial gaps develop in the capillaries shortly after burning and this results in exudation of plasma from the surface of the burn and into the interstitial spaces. Changes in plasma oncotic pressure and hydrostatic pressure in the tissues alter the rates of loss and produce the final clinical picture. In patients with cutaneous burns of greater than 30% of the body surface area, oedema also develops in non-burned tissue after approximately eight hours. Smaller endothelial gaps are demonstrable in non-burned tissues and oedema formation is thought to be related to hypoproteinaemia.

Because of these sequential alterations in plasma loss, most burns resuscitation protocols are divided into periods from the time of burning. In the A&E department, it is the early losses which are important and it is only necessary to memorize the likely fluid requirement for the first eight hours after burning. Because the patient is initially treated in the A&E department, it is the responsibility of those treating him to remember that all protocols are described as if treatment commences immediately after burning. There may well be some catching up required for the untreated period prior to admission to hospital. If this catching up is not addressed in the A&E department the period of hypovolaemia suffered by the patient may be far longer than is necessary. The protocols are only intended as a guide to the volume of fluid required and the volumes given may have to be adjusted to ensure a minimum urine output of 0.5 ml/kg body weight/hour, a pulse rate of about 120 beats/minute and normal acid-base balance. It has been clearly demonstrated in burned patients that the subsequent development and number of multiple organ failures can be directly correlated to the severity of shock. There is no doubt that hypovolaemia and tissue hypoxia are as important in the burned patient as they are in the non-burned patient who is severely injured.

# How much of which type of fluid for resuscitation?

As for the severely injured patient, there is considerable debate as to the optimum fluid for plasma replacement after burning and the biggest differences are found in the parts of the protocol relating to the first eight hours after injury (Table 2.3.1). In practice, all the protocols have been demonstrated to be effective in large numbers of patients. The A&E doctor may find it helpful to understand the thoughts which are behind the various protocols.

The protocols fall into three broad groups. In the first group, isotonic crystalloid solutions are given in the first 24 hours because they are effective and it is claimed that

**Table 2.3.1 Fluid replacement regimes for cutaneous burns**

| Formula | Fluid type | Total volume for first 8 hours |
|---------|-----------|-------------------------------|
| Muir and Barclay[1] | Plasma | 1.0 ml/kg/% burn |
| Birmingham Accident Hospital[2] | Plasma and Dextran 110 alternately in equal volumes | 70 ml/% burn |
| Parkland[3] | Ringers lactate | 2 ml/kg/% burn |
| Brooke[3] | Ringers lactate Plasma | 0.5 ml/kg/% burn 0.25 ml/kg/% burn |

1. Muir, I.F.K., Barclay, T.L. and Settle, J.A.D. (1987). *Burns and their Treatment*, 3rd edn. London: Butterworths.
2. Cason, J.S. (1981). *Treatment of Burns*. London: Chapman and Hall.
3. Pruitt, B.A. (1978). Fluid and electrolyte replacement in the burned patient. *Surg. Clin. N. Amer.*, **58**, 1291–1312.

capillary permeability is such that all fluids will leak out of the circulation so that it is unnecessary to replace proteins at this stage. In the second group, colloid solutions are given in the first 24 hours because plasma is being lost, plasma osmotic pressure is said to be better maintained by the transfusion of colloidal solutions and hypoproteinaemia is thought to be the cause of oedema in non-burned tissues. In the third group, crystalloid and colloid solutions are given and the arguments of both the crystalloid and colloid protagonists are cited.

Other factors such as cost and the fear of blood-borne infection are also important. Crystalloid solutions are cheapest, but when colloids are administered the precise choice of colloid often reflects the cost of the solutions rather than their physiological properties.

Hypertonic saline has also been used successfully. It has many of the advantages of colloid solutions but is cheaper and is free of the risk of infection. It is also claimed that it minimizes oedema formation. There have been reports of dangerously high serum osmolarity and sodium levels following its use and a safe protocol has not yet been published. It is probable that hypertonic saline will eventually find a place in the resuscitation of burned patients and that it will be used in A&E departments.

# The significance of hypoxia during definitive management

In the burned patient, the causation of hypoxia is usually fairly obvious and is due to chemical injury to the lower airways, profound shock or, rarely, pneumothorax, haemothorax or inhalation of gastric contents. Regular monitoring of arterial blood gases and other parameters of respiratory function will enable prompt detection and correction of any deterioration.

In the burned patient, it is the presence of apparently adequate levels of arterial oxygenation which may be dangerous if monitoring data is accepted at face value. Pulse oximeters and standard arterial blood gas analysers fail to distinguish between normally oxygenated haemoglobin and carboxyhaemoglobin. This problem has been highlighted already and the need for additional oxygen has been stressed. It is vital to interpret information from these monitoring devices in the light of measured carboxyhaemoglobin levels.

In cyanide poisoning, arterial oxygenation may also be normal. In this instance, it is the intracellular energy mechanisms which are paralysed such that oxygen cannot be effectively utilized.

In both types of poisoning, the measurement of arterial oxygenation will not assist in the management of the problem. It is possible to gain some idea of the severity of tissue hypoxia by measuring the base deficit and blood lactate levels. The frequency of combined carbon monoxide and cyanide poisoning has already been noted. Furthermore, hypovolaemia also causes tissue hypoxia. In the A&E department, it is impossible to identify the relative contributions of hypovolaemia and each type of poison to the level of tissue hypoxia. In practice, all that can be done is to ensure that maximal concentrations of oxygen are administered to all patients at risk, that meticulous fluid replacement is commenced, that the diagnosis of carbon monoxide poisoning is made and that if there are other significant clues to the presence of cyanide poisoning, that an antidote is given.

# *Reassessment and monitoring the response to treatment*

In the burned patient, it is essential to continue monitoring the patient's response to treatment for the first 48 hours. In all probability, the secondary survey will have identified the exact extent of the cutaneous burn and the presence of inhalational injury. It is unlikely that potentially significant injuries will have been missed but it may not be possible, in the A&E department, to predict how quickly laryngeal swelling will occur or the time of onset of bronchospasm and its ultimate severity. Vigilant monitoring will provide clues which may be helpful to the doctors who take over the care of the patient in the same hospital or to the A&E doctors if the decision is made to transfer the patient to a Regional Burns Unit. In the latter case, it is the responsibility of the transferring doctor to ensure that all developments during the journey are anticipated and prepared for. While it is acceptable to closely monitor the patient with potential airway swelling if he is remaining in the same hospital, it is often more appropriate to perform prophylactic endotracheal intubation if transfer is planned.

The problems of non-invasive monitoring have already been described. Invasive monitoring is rarely required. It is probably better to leave the decision about the desirability of an arterial line to the Burns Unit doctors unless clear hospital protocols for their insertion exist. The indications for the use of a pulmonary artery flotation catheter in the A&E department are limited as the patient is usually transferred rapidly within the hospital or to another institution. The use of such a catheter may be contemplated if the patient has a pulmonary injury and myocardial failure. In the presence of pulmonary injury it is essential to avoid fluid overload as this exacerbates oedema formation and may lead rapidly to the development of the adult respiratory distress syndrome. It is, however, usual for patients with combined cutaneous and respiratory burns to require up to 20% more fluid during resuscitation than the patient with an equivalent cutaneous burn without pulmonary injury. The likelihood of gross overload occurring in the A&E department is, therefore, remote. It is rare for myocardial failure to cause significant problems in the A&E department.

# The provision of analgesia and sedation

The most severely burned patients are often least in need of pain relief as full thickness burns are painless. In the presence of painful partial thickness burns or erythema, pain relief must be provided. Usually Entonox or an opiate infusion is the most appropriate. These and other methods of pain relief have been described on p. 76.

It is extremely unusual for a burned patient to be agitated without a good reason. The causes listed for injured patients in Table 1.3.3 (p. 81) are equally applicable to burned patients and sedative drugs should only be administered in the circumstances described on pp. 80–82.

# Emergency surgery and anaesthesia in the resuscitation room

Anaesthesia and surgery are rarely necessary in the emergency room. An emergency tracheostomy may be required if total airway obstruction has already occurred and the anesthetist has failed to pass an endotracheal tube. Gross hypoxia will already have caused unconsciousness. It is sufficient for the anaesthetist to supply oxygen as soon as the airway is secured. The surgeon may choose to use an adrenaline and local anaesthetic solution to reduce bleeding and this provides sufficient anaesthesia.

Delay in admission to hospital with circumferential full thickness burns to the chest or a limb may pose a threat to life or limb. Releasing incisions can be life or limb saving but anaesthesia is almost always unnecessary (pp. 137–138).

# Specific burn injuries of importance to the anaesthetist

## *Smoke inhalation*

Smoke inhalation may cause a variety of problems, the nature of which depends on the characteristics of the smoke which has been inhaled. They may be classified into thermal effects, chemical effects, mechanical effects and systemic poisoning ( Table 2.4.1). Most of these have been described individually in foregoing sections. This may have led the reader to believe that each problem occurs in isolation. Unfortunately, this is not true. Most patients with smoke inhalation have suffered more than one effect.

**Thermal effects.**   These are manifest as burns to the mouth, oropharynx and larynx. Because the mouth is wet with saliva, excess heat is dissipated by evaporation so the burns are rarely full thickness. The main problem is swelling, which

**Table 2.4.1 The effects of smoke inhalation**

| | | |
|---|---|---|
| Thermal damage | Oropharyngeal swelling | Hot smoke |
| | Laryngeal swelling | Hot smoke |
| | Tracheal swelling | Superheated steam |
| Chemical damage | Irritation and bronchospasm | Ammonia, sulphur dioxide, chlorine, aldehydes, phosphorus, oxides of nitrogen |
| | Alveolar capillary damage and pulmonary oedema | Aldehydes, phosphorus, oxides of nitrogen, acrolein |
| Mechanical obstruction | Soot | Ammonia, sulphur dioxide, hydrochloric acid, acrolein |
| | Sloughing of airway mucosa | |
| Systemic poisoning | Decreased oxygen-carrying capacity | Carbon monoxide |
| | Inhibition of cytochrome oxidase | Cyanide |

can cause airway obstruction. Electrical burns to the mouth can occur. Commonly they are seen in children who have attempted to chew an electrical cable. The burns are usually full thickness and have involved muscle. Swelling can be extensive and may affect the airway particularly if the tongue swells excessively. Early intubation is sometimes indicated and may be difficult because of the full thickness burn around the mouth.

Inhaled gases have already cooled by the time they have passed through the larynx. Further evaporation cools the gases in the trachea, which is an efficient dissipator of heat. Unless super-heated steam is inhaled, it is unusual to see thermal burns below the level of the glottis.

**Chemical effects**.  Patients involved in house and vehicle fires are particularly prone to chemical burns of the lower airway. Polyvinyl chloride, polyurethane, Teflon and Melamine release a variety of toxic products which include hydrogen chloride, phosgene, chlorine, formaldehyde, ammonia and hydrogen cyanide which are themselves toxic and form acids when dissolved in water. Wood and paper produce acrolein which is also injurious to the airways.

Chemical burns to the airways cause oedema and, if severe, damage to the alveoli. The clinical picture is similar to that seen in pulmonary contusion and the management is similar (pp. 96–98).

**Mechanical effects**. Carbon particles contained in smoke may, if present in large quantities, cause obstruction of the smaller airways and alveoli. Aggressive physiotherapy, supplemented in severe cases by bronchoscopy, will help to remove the carbon.

In addition, many inhaled gases such as phosgene, chlorine and ammonia are irritant to the airways and may provoke bronchospasm. The clinical picture is similar to that of an attack of acute asthma and is treated similarly (pp. 204–206). Highly soluble toxic substances such as ammonia, sulphur dioxide, hydrochloric acid and acrolein cause sloughing of the bronchial mucosa and swelling of the bronchial blood vessels. The latter effect may contribute to the development of pulmonary oedema.

**Poisoning**. Carbon monoxide and cyanide poisoning may occur, with or without the inhalation of carbonaceous smoke and facial burns and are discussed in the following pages.

# Carbon monoxide poisoning

Carbon monoxide poisoning is commonly associated with smoke inhalation but may occur in other situations. Inhalation of exhaust fumes, heating systems with faulty ventilation and leakage of household, but not natural, gas are well recognized causes of carbon monoxide poisoning.

Blood levels of up to 0.7% are normal and occur as a result of endogenous production. Levels of 2% in non-smokers and 6% in smokers are common when these people live in a heavily polluted urban environment.

**Pathophysiology**.   Carbon monoxide binds to iron molecules in haemoglobin and its affinity for it is 200 to 250 times that of oxygen. This means that it will displace oxygen from haemoglobin. Carbon monoxide binding to haemoglobin also induces allosteric changes in the remaining oxygen binding sites which increases the affinity of haemoglobin for oxygen. This causes a distortion in the shape of the oxygen dissociation curve as well as shifting it to the left. All these changes reduce the availability of oxygen to the tissues.

Carbon monoxide may also bind with other haem proteins, such as cytochrome oxidase, and inhibit cellular respiration in the same way as cyanide. There is still some debate as to the significance of this effect in pure carbon monoxide poisoning but there is animal evidence to suggest a synergistic hypoxic effect when carbon monoxide and cyanide poisoning occur together.

**Clinical symptoms and signs**.   These are immensely variable and depend on the severity and duration of exposure and the patient's general physical fitness. Chronic exposure causes headache, fatigue, difficulty in thinking, dizziness, paraesthesia, chest pain, palpitations, visual disturbance, nausea, diarrhoea and abdominal pain, all of which may be mistaken for other conditions.

Acute poisoning is easier to recognize because the history will suggest the diagnosis. Even so, symptoms and signs may vary enormously and do not correlate well with subsequent estimations of carboxyhaemoglobin level. Generally, blood concentrations of less than 10% are not associated with symptoms, concentrations of 10–30% may cause only headache and mild dyspnoea and concentrations above 60%

cause convulsions, coma and cardiorespiratory arrest (Table 2.2.2, p. 127).

Acute life-threatening problems from carbon monoxide poisoning include cardiorespiratory arrest, loss of airway control due to coma or convulsions and dysrhythmias secondary to myocardial infarction or ischaemia. Days or weeks after severe poisoning, hypoxic damage may be manifest as severe neurological defects such as prolonged coma or hemiplegia, hepatic failure, renal failure or intestinal gangrene.

**Management**. Emergency management consists of administering 100% oxygen. If the airway is compromised, endotracheal intubation is indicated and will guarantee the delivery of high concentrations of oxygen. If endotracheal intubation is not required, a tightly fitting face mask must be used. The plastic face masks commonly used to administer oxygen tend to be loose fitting and rarely deliver oxygen at a concentration of above 60%. The administration of 100% oxygen reduces the elimination half life of carbon monoxide to 40 minutes from 240 minutes if the patient is left to breathe room air.

Supportive measures may be required if the patient is comatose. Controlled mechanical ventilation and mannitol may help to control cerebral oedema. Corticosteroids have been advocated but are of dubious value. Dantrolene sodium has been used successfully to control muscle rigidity and hyperpyrexia.

Hyperbaric oxygen pressurized to two atmospheres reduces the elimination half life of carbon monoxide to 20 minutes. It is only available in a few locations and its benefits are still unclear. It is probable that it reduces the duration of coma and the severity of long-term morbidity, particularly neuropsychiatric sequelae, even if it is not given until several hours after poisoning. It has been suggested that hyperbaric oxygen should be considered urgently if there has been an episode of unconsciousness, definite neurological signs, cardiac complications, for pregnant women and for all patients with carboxyhaemoglobin levels above 40%, regardless of the symptoms.

## FURTHER READING

Anon. (1988). Treatment of carbon monoxide poisoning. *Drugs Therap. Bull.*, **26**, 77–79.

Meredith, T. and Vale, A. (1988). Carbon monoxide poisoning. *Br. Med. J.*, **296**, 77–78.

# *Cyanide poisoning*

Cyanide poisoning, contrary to popular opinion, does not always cause immediate death. Blood levels of cyanide of 0.2 mg/l are toxic and levels above 1 mg/l are fatal. Poisoning may be due to inhalation as a result of fire or an industrial accident or ingestion of cyanide compounds used by farmers and foresters for killing rabbits. Dermal and occular absorption can also occur. Burning polyurethane, polyacrylonitrile, styrene and wool produce cyanide fumes. Combined carbon monoxide and cyanide poisoning may be responsible of one third of deaths from house fires.

**Pathophysiology.**   Cyanide combines with the ferric iron of the mitochondrial enzyme cytochrome oxidase and prevents oxygen binding, thus inhibiting cellular respiration and causing severe tissue hypoxia.

**Clinical symptoms and signs.**   Mild poisoning causes non-specific symptoms of anxiety, headache, tachypnoea and vomiting. Diagnosis, in the absence of a suggestive history, is difficult. Severe poisoning causes hypotension, pulmonary oedema, coma and respiratory depression. Blood cyanide levels can be measured but the results are not immediately available. A retrospective diagnosis can be made, but in the emergency situation the medical staff must make the diagnosis on other evidence such as a persistent, unexplained, metabolic acidosis or raised serum lactate levels, both of which are indicators of severe tissue hypoxia

**Management**. Initially supportive treatment to restore the airway, ensure adequate ventilation, optimize the circulating blood volume and support the failing myocardium is indicated. One hundred per cent oxygen should always be administered in order to ensure that as much oxygen is available to the tissues as possible. Oxygen has also been shown to increase rhodanase activity, which may be helpful. Hyperbaric oxygen has not been shown to be beneficial.

After initial resuscitation has been started, consideration may be given to the administration of a cyanide antidote. It has been suggested that treatment should be given if the carboyxhaemoglobin level is greater than 15% because the two types of poisoning so often occur together. Several cyanide antidotes are available, but in the absence of a positive diagnosis may be as dangerous as cyanide poisoning itself.

Inhaled amyl nitrate or intravenous sodium nitrite have been advocated because they produce methaemoglobin which can compete with and displace cyanide from binding sites on the cytochrome oxidase molecule. These drugs should be used with caution because a high concentration of methaemoglobin can also cause hypoxia and all nitrites may cause vasodilatation and severe hypotension.

An intravenous dose of 300 mg cobalt edetate will effectively chelate cyanide but may cause hypotension, hypertension, cardiac arrhythmias or a severe anaphylactoid reaction. In excess, cobalt may bind to cytochrome oxidase and prevent oxygen binding in a similar way to cyanide.

Mitochondrial rhodanase causes dissociation of the cytochrome oxidase and cyanide complex by transferring sulphur from thiosulphate to cyanide. Thiocyanate, which is harmless, is formed. Sulphur can be provided in the form of sodium thiosulphate administered intravenously in a dose of 12.5 g in a 50 ml volume over 10 minutes. Sodium thiosulphate is free of serious side effects but may not be effective in cyanide poisoning because it penetrates cell membranes far more slowly than cyanide and there is a delay before effective tissue levels are reached. Hydroxocobalamin, administered intravenously in a dose of 4 g, is effective and is non-toxic except for occasional mild allergic reactions. Its use is limited only by cost and the difficulty of obtaining a suitable high dose preparation.

# PART THREE

# Life-threatening problems of medical and surgical emergencies

Theoretical aspects

# *Hypoxia, hypovolaemia and myocardial failure*

In recent years, there has been much debate about the high preventable mortality rate following major trauma. The Royal College of Surgeons report on 'The Management of Patients with Major Injuries' noted that only 1% of patients admitted to hospital through the A&E department had major injuries. The majority of admissions through the A&E department are for medical and surgical conditions or for minor traumatic injuries. It is therefore surprising that scant attention has been paid to the possibility that some medical and surgical deaths in the A&E department may also be preventable.

In 1984, Shalley and Cross studied 488 deaths occurring in a busy A&E department over a five-year period. They found that 87% of deaths were due to medical causes, 8% due to surgical causes and the remainder were due to the effects of serious injury. It is notable that all of the deaths medical and surgical would have caused difficulties with the airway, breathing or circulation and were associated with hypoxia, hypovolaemia or myocardial failure. There were preventable deaths although these were not quantified. These deaths were due to failure to protect the airway and hence pulmonary inhalation of gastric contents, failure to treat hypovolaemia with sufficient speed and quantities of blood and failure to recognize that breathing difficulties were due to a pneumothorax.

These findings suggest that an approach to the management of medical and surgical emergencies similar to that advocated for major trauma and burns has merit. A rapid primary survey to identify airway, breathing and circulatory insufficiency should be followed by life-saving measures. When resuscitation has been started, the secondary survey can be performed to identify, first, pathophysiological abnormalities requiring treatment and, second, to come to a diagnosis. When patients have sustained burn or non-burn injuries, one of the important reasons for reassessing the patient after definitive treatment that has been given is to identify injuries which may have been missed. The fact that in medical and surgical emergencies a single diagnosis should be sought to explain all the symptoms does not alter the need to reassess the patient once definitive treatment has been commenced. The treatment in progress may be inadequate or the patient may have developed new symptoms and signs which may change the original diagnosis.

## FURTHER READING

Shalley, M.J. and Cross A.B. (1984). Which patients are likely to die in an accident and emergency department? *Br. Med. J.*, **289**, 419–421.

# The pathophysiological effects of medical and surgical disease

Hypoxia, hypovolaemia and myocardial failure are the major life-threatening problems suffered by medical and surgical patients. In medical patients, hypoxia and myocardial failure are by far the commonest problems whereas surgical patients are more similar to patients with multiple injuries and burns because the most significant problem is often hypovolaemia.

Although the evidence is less well documented, there is little reason to suppose that the effects of tissue hypoxia are any less important in medical and surgical patients than they are in severely injured ,patients. There is no doubt that medical and surgical patients, being treated for sepsis in the intensive care unit, develop organ failure in the same way as patients with major injuries and burns. Prompt and effective treatment in the A&E department may well reduce the incidence and severity of subsequent complications.

# Medical and surgical problems which may affect cellular oxygenation

The general principles of cellular oxygenation described on pp. 11–17 are applicable to medical and surgical emergencies as is an identical pathophysiological approach to the identification of problems.

**Inhaled oxygen concentration**.   High inspired oxygen concentrations are beneficial to all patients who are hypoxic, hypovolaemic or in myocardial failure. The only exceptions to this rule are patients with an acute exacerbation of chronic bronchitis who are dependent on hypoxia for their respiratory drive. These patients should be given the maximum concentration of inspired oxygen consistent with continued respiratory effort.

**Transfer of oxygen to the trachea and bronchial tree**. Transfer of oxygen to the bronchial tree is dependent on patency of the upper airway and trachea and on adequate excursion of the chest wall. The causes of upper airway obstruction are listed in Table 3.1.1. Poor respiratory excursion of the chest wall may be due to inadequate cerebral control, pain due to intrathoracic or abdominal pathology or diaphragmatic splinting by the abdominal contents. Abdominal swelling may be due to massive haemorrhage, bowel distention, ascites, or massive hepatomegaly.

**Transfer of oxygen from the bronchial tree to the alveolar capillary membrane**. Pneumothorax, haemothorax, pleural effusion and emphysema will cause external compression of the lungs and reduce expansion of the alveoli. Gas flow to the alveoli may be reduced by inhaled substances such as

**Table 3.1.1 Causes of upper airway obstruction in medical and surgical patients**

1.  Loss of protective airway reflexes
    (a) Cerebrovascular accidents and neurological disorders
    (b) Alcohol and drugs
    (c) Hypoxia
    (d) Hypovolaemia

2.  Laryngeal or tracheal obstruction
    (a) Swelling: (i) allergy, (ii) epiglottitis,
    (iii) oropharyngeal infection, (iv) radiotherapy
    (b) Tumour
    (c) Hereditary angioneurotic oedema

3.  Foreign bodies
    (a) Solid food
    (b) False teeth
    (c) Miscellaneous objects, e.g. peanuts, coins, chewing gum

blood, vomit or foreign bodies, intrinsic narrowing of the airways by bronchospasm or tumours and extrinsic narrowing of the airways due to tumours. Infected sputum and pulmonary oedema may obscure the alveolar membrane and prevent oxygen reaching the alveolar capillary membrane.

**Transfer of oxygen across the alveolar capillary membrane to the blood**.   Transfer of oxygen across the alveolar membrane may be reduced by excessive sputum or by pulmonary oedema. Oedema may also widen the interstitial space between the alveolar and capillary membrane. In addition to low flow states due to relative hypovolaemia, absolute hypovolaemia and myocardial failure, pulmonary perfusion may be significantly reduced in the medical patient by a large pulmonary embolus. Chronic anaemia is a more common problem in medical and surgical patients than in injured and burned patients because the onset of the diseases leading to emergency admission is often insidious. It can significantly reduce the oxygen-carrying capacity of the blood and contribute to tissue hypoxia.

**Circulation of the blood to the tissues**.   Blood flow to the tissues may be reduced by absolute hypovolaemia. Acute blood loss is seen in patients with bleeding peptic ulcers, bleeding oesophageal varices and with ruptured aortic aneurysms. Plasma may be lost in large volumes into the wall of obstructed bowel. Dehydration due to prolonged vomiting, profuse diarrhoea or heat exposure will also reduce the circulating blood volume. Relative hypovolaemia occurs if there has been vasodilatation due to sepsis or a severe allergic reaction. Myocardial function may be impaired by an acute ischaemic episode, some dysrhythmias, myocardial infarction, cardiomyopathy and sepsis. Rarely a spontaneous pneumothorax may tension. The effects of hypovolaemia and myocardial impairment are identical to the effects of the same problems in severely injured patients (pp. 43–48).

**Transfer of oxygen to the capillaries**.   The problems are similar to those seen in severely injured patients. The toxic metabolites released by injury, shock and sepsis have been less well studied in the acute phase of medical and surgical emergencies. It is known, however, that patients with acute pancreatitis behave similarly to severely injured patients. It is probable that complement, arachidonic acid metabolites and free oxygen radicals are also released by emergency medical and surgical conditions with potentially devastating effects.

# *Treatment goals*

The goal should be to minimize and, if possible, prevent tissue hypoxia. The goals are identical to those described for severely injured and burned patients. They are:

1. Ensure adequate oxygenation and ventilation of the respiratory tract.
2. Restore the circulating blood volume to normal.
3. Reverse vasoconstriction.
4. Optimize myocardial contractility.
5. Optimize arterial red cell content to facilitate oxygen transport and capillary blood flow.
6. Normalize erythrocyte oxygen affinity.

# Practical aspects and definitive management

## *Ethical considerations*

The study performed by Shalley and Cross (p. 167) showed that 6% of patients dying in the A&E department were suffering from carcinomatosis. This is greater than the number dying from severe injuries. It is noted with sadness that relatives have to rely on hospital care in terminal illness, and that it is undignified and distressing for patients in this category to die in a busy A&E department.

In terminal illness, resuscitative measures are usually inappropriate. The patient, in consultation with his relatives, will usually already have decided the extent and nature of care that he wishes to receive. It is, however, essential that patients with terminal illness die with dignity and in comfort. The anaesthetist has a wide range of skills relating to the management of pain relief and sedation. These should be utilized to the full.

Sometimes, resuscitation is commenced before the terminal nature of the disease is recognized. Anaesthetists and their A&E colleagues should have an agreed protocol for the management of these unfortunate patients.

# The causes and diagnosis of upper airway obstruction

The causes of upper airway obstruction in medical and surgical emergencies are listed in Table 3.1.1 (p. 169). The signs of upper airway obstruction are similar to those seen in severely injured and burned patients. The methods of diagnosing airway obstruction are identical for all patients. The reader is referred to pp. 20–21 for a description of the methods available.

# General management principles for upper airway obstruction and methods of securing the airway

**If in doubt, secure the airway**. In medical and surgical patients, the commonest cause of upper airway obstruction is loss of consciousness. The airway not only becomes obstructed when the tongue falls backwards but also the reduction in the level of consciousness obtunds the protective laryngeal and carinal reflexes. The risk of aspiration of stomach contents into the patient's lungs is significant. If there is any doubt about the patency or security of the airway, it should be protected. The methods used are identical to those already described (pp. 24–50).

In medical and surgical patients, mechanical obstruction to the upper airway may be due to foreign bodies such as false teeth, laryngeal oedema as a result of allergy or radiotherapy to the oropharynx or larynx or due to swellings resulting from abscesses or tumours. In these patients, there is a danger that the doctor will be unable to secure the airway by endotracheal intubation. This may be because of the primary pathology or because instrumentation of the airway has aggravated swelling or caused bleeding. If there is time, it is usual to have a surgeon standing by so that an emergency tracheostomy can be performed if intubation fails. In some centres, it is customary to move the patient to an operating theatre before attempting endotracheal intubation. These are wise precautions but the patient may become severely hypoxic if there is a delay before the airway is secured. If intubation fails and until a formal tracheostomy is created, the cricothyrotomy is an ideal method of establishing a temporary airway in these patients. The presence of a surgeon should not distract the anaesthetist from his prime duty, which is to maintain oxygenation *at all times*.

Normal anatomical variants, the risk of pulmonary aspiration of stomach contents, massive pulmonary haemorrhage or oedema, and the clenched jaw are all problems which may make endotracheal intubation more difficult and can turn a difficult intubation into an impossible one. They have already been discussed on pp. 30–33.

# The causes, diagnosis and general management principles for respiratory insufficiency

Respiratory insufficiency has four major causes. These are inadequate or inappropriate movement of the chest wall, inadequate lung expansion, abnormal respiratory drive and impaired gas exchange. There may be a variety of causes for these abnormalities which are summarized in Table 3.2.1. The approach to diagnosis is similar to that described for patients with major injuries (pp. 34–38).

**Inadequate or inappropriate movement of the chest wall**. Inadequate movement of the chest wall is most commonly due to underlying pulmonary pathology such as pneumothorax, pleural effusion or consolidation due to infection. Sometimes it can be due to pain secondary to pleurisy. Having observed the abnormal or inappropriate movement, percussion and auscultation of the chest should confirm the diagnosis. Inadequate movement of the chest wall is rarely due to neurological problems such as disseminated sclerosis, the Guillain–Barré syndrome or acute poliomyelitis. A neurological examination of the patient will reveal other abnormalities which should give a clue to the diagnosis.

**Inadequate lung expansion**. This may be due to inadequate chest wall movement, compression of the lungs by air, serous fluid or pus and by decreased airflow in the upper or lower airways due to partial or complete obstruction. Again, the diagnosis may be made by percussion and auscultation of the chest. If there is time, a chest X-ray may confirm the presence of air or fluid in the pleural cavity.

**Abnormal respiratory drive**. This may be due to metabolic or brain stem abnormalities. In the medical patient,

175

**Table 3.2.1 The causes of respiratory insufficiency in medical and surgical patients**

---

1. Upper airway obstruction
   Table 3.1.1 (p. 169)

2. Inadequate or inappropriate chest wall excursion
   (a) Pleuritic pain
   (b) Peripheral nerve abnormalities, e.g. Guillain–Barré syndrome, Myaesthenia gravis, disseminated sclerosis, poliomyelitis

3. Inadequate lung expansion
   (a) Inadequate chest wall excursion
   (b) Spontaneous pneumothorax
   (c) Pleural effusion
   (d) Infective consolidation
   (e) Pulmonary collapse secondary to sputum plug, tumour or foreign body
   (f) Bronchospasm

4. Abnormal respiratory drive
   (a) Coma (Table 3.2.5, p. 188)
   (b) Hypovolaemia
   (c) Hypoxia

5. Impaired gas exchange
   (a) Pulmonary collapse
   (b) Pulmonary oedema
   (c) Pulmonary aspiration of blood or stomach contents
   (d) Pulmonary embolism
   (e) Inadequate pulmonary perfusion secondary to hypovolaemia or myocardial failure

---

hyperglycaemic coma, cerebrovascular accidents and sub-arachnoid haemorrhage are common causes of abnormal respiratory drive. In the surgical patient, an acute rise in intracranial pressure secondary to haemorrhage into a cerebral tumour may cause respiratory abnormalities. Rarely, hepatic encephalopathy, a uraemic crisis or the acute onset of septicaemia cause abnormalities of respiratory drive. The diagnosis and treatment of these problems is described elsewhere.

**Impaired gas exchange**. Unless the patient has inhaled gastric contents, impaired gas exchange due to occlusion of the alveoli will be due to pulmonary oedema or infected sputum. A history from the ambulance staff or relatives may give a clue to the diagnosis, a sample of sputum can be diagnostic and auscultation and chest X-ray will confirm the provisional diagnosis.

Inadequate pulmonary blood flow secondary to pulmonary embolism, absolute hypovolaemia or myocardial failure may impair oxygen uptake by the circulation. The diagnosis of these problems is described elsewhere.

**General principles of management**. These have already been described on pp. 38–40 and may be summarized as follows. All patients benefit from oxygen administered through a face mask or endotracheal tube. Analgesia should be given if required, lung expansion promoted by drainage of the pleural cavity, vigorous physiotherapy to clear secretions aided if necessary by a cricothyroidotomy, diuretics to reduce oedema, bronchodilators to correct bronchospasm, bronchoscopy to remove solid obstructions such as foreign bodies or inhaled food and, if all these fail or the patient is in extremis, controlled mechanical ventilation. If the respiratory drive is impaired or chest wall movement is limited by neurological problems, controlled mechanical ventilation is indicated. This should be started in conjunction with definitive treatments such as insulin for hyperglycaemic coma. For chronic bronchitics with acute or chronic infection, a respiratory stimulant such as doxapram may buy time and avoid the need for mechanical ventilation. Impaired gas exchange may be treated by physiotherapy to clear infected secretions, diuretics to reduce pulmonary oedema and, in severe cases, controlled mechanical ventilation. Circulatory insufficiency should be treated with intravenous colloids for hypovolaemia and inotropes and vasodilators for myocardial failure.

# Difficulties in the management of respiratory insufficiency

The problems encountered with patients with major injuries (pp. 40–43) are not specific to this group of patients and are equally applicable to patients with medical and surgical conditions.

**The decision to commence ventilation**.   As with the severely injured patient, ventilation should be commenced immediately if the patient is grossly cyanosed even though oxygen is being given and if respiratory effort is absent or grossly inadequate. In all other cases, the response to treatment should be closely monitored and ventilation initiated if there is a deterioration in respiratory function in spite of appropriate treatment.

**Inability to ventilate the lungs**.   In addition to the problems mentioned on pp. 41–42, inability to ventilate the lungs in the medical patient may be due to severe bronchospasm. Bronchodilators should be given (Table 3.2.2) and the

**Table 3.2.2 The treatment of bronchospasm in adults**

| First | Oxygen by mask |
| | Sit the patient up |
| Then | Salbutamol 5–10 mg nebulized |
| | Ipratropium bromide 0.5 mg nebulized |
| If no improvement | Hydrocortisone 200 mg intravenously |
| | Aminophylline 250 mg intravenously slowly |
| | (contraindicated if patient has already taken |
| | theophylline derivatives) |
| | *or* |
| | Terbutaline 0.5 mg subcutaneously |
| Still no improvement | Consider controlled mechanical ventilation |
| | Aminophylline infusion 500 mg over 4 hours |

patient manually ventilated, allowing plenty of time for each expiratory breath.

**Inability to achieve adequate arterial oxygenation**.   Assuming that the oxygen delivery system is functioning correctly and the patient's cardiovascular status has been normalized, this problem is rare and usually carries a poor prognosis. Inadequate arterial oxygenation may be due to severe primary pulmonary pathology, an undiagnosed pneumothorax secondary to controlled mechanical ventilation or due to a large pulmonary embolus for which the only effective treatment may be surgical removal.

# The causes and diagnosis of cardiovascular insufficiency

The six major causes of cardiovascular collapse described for patients with major injuries (Table 1.2.2, p. 43) are also applicable to medical and surgical emergencies although the frequency of their occurrence is different and the underlying pathological causes are also different. Cardiovascular collapse can be diagnosed if two major pulses are impalpable.

**Major haemorrhage**.   With the exception of patients with a ruptured aortic aneurysm, it is rare for major haemorrhage to cause cardiac arrest in medical and surgical emergencies who reach the A&E department alive. Bleeding from oesophageal varices, obstetric emergencies and bleeding ulcers may be heavy but prompt fluid administration should avert life-threatening cardiovascular collapse.

**Cardiac arrest**.   This is usually due to a massive myocardial infarction, massive pulmonary embolism or to a dysrhythmia which impairs cardiac output. Severe septicaemia may also cause a cardiac arrest due to the myocardial depressant effects of endotoxins. Cardiac arrest in septic patients can be difficult to treat unless the vasodilator effect of the endotoxins and the capillary damage and fluid loss which they also cause are recognized and treated. Viral myocarditis can cause cardiac arrest and is often subclinical until this catastrophic event occurs.

**Myocardial failure**. Myocardial failure is usually due to severe ischaemia which either diminishes myocardial muscle contractility at the time of the collapse or has caused previous damage which makes the patient susceptible to dysrhythmias which are incompatible with normal cardiac function. The ischaemic episode may occur as a result of coronary artery spasm which reduces myocardial blood flow or as a consequence of severe respiratory failure or arrest.

Overdose of certain drugs, particularly the tricyclic antidepressants can cause life-threatening dysrhythmias. Rarely, myocardial failure may be due to cardiac tamponade secondary to infection or cancer. The accumulation of fluid in the pericardial sac is slow and normally produces symptoms leading to the correct diagnosis and appropriate treatment before the critical volume, which causes cardiovascular collapse, is reached. In rare instances, however, the diagnosis may not be made until the time of admission to the A&E department. Similarly, constrictive cardiomyopathy has an insidious onset, but again the correct diagnosis may not have been made.

**Cardiac tamponade**. See above under myocardial failure and p. 45.

**Tension pneumothorax**. Spontaneous pneumothorax is a relatively common occurrence whose symptoms are not always taken seriously by the patient. There is, therefore, the potential for a tension pneumothorax to develop and to cause cardiovascular collapse within a relatively short period of time in a previously fit patient with no previous history of illness. The diagnosis and management are discussed on pp. 45 and 49.

**Massive cerebral damage**.    Any major intracranial event can cause cardiac arrest. This may be due to a specific lesion of the brain stem such as the development of a tumour, an infarct or haemorrhage or because of coning of the brain stem through the foramen magnum as a result of a rise in intracranial pressure due to haemorrhage or swelling.

# *General management principles for cardiovascular insufficiency*

The management of cardiovascular collapse depends on the diagnosis. Although in medical and surgical patients hypovolaemia is not so frequently the cause of collapse as it is in the severely injured or burned patient, it is still vital to secure venous access as rapidly as possible. With the exception of bleeding from a dissecting thoracic aortic aneurysm, the site of venous access is less critical than in the severely injured patient and a single site of access above the diaphragm is often sufficient. Although central venous pressure catheters are unsuitable for the rapid transfusion of fluid, they can provide a useful route for injecting drugs to stimulate the myocardium.

**Hypovolaemia**.    All patients should be given oxygen. Fluids should be transfused rapidly. The precise regime is less important than the speed and accuracy with which it is administered. If the diagnosis is in doubt, repeated challenges with 200 ml of fluid should be given. Careful monitoring is essential to detect when the administration of fluid no longer produces an increase in central venous pressure accompanied by a reduction in heart rate and a rise in blood pressure. The fluid regime used for injured patients (pp. 48–49) is suitable for hypovolaemic medical and surgical patients who are bleeding. In other types of hypovolaemia, the type of fluid administered should be chosen according to the type of loss. In septicaemia, colloids and sometimes blood are appropriate. For bowel obstruction, crystalloids and colloids are preferable. Dehydration responds well to crystalloids. Additional electrolytes should be given as indicated.

**Cardiac arrest**. Having established that cardiac arrest has occurred, the patency of the airway and adequacy of breathing must also be checked. If necessary, endotracheal intubation and ventilation of the lungs must form part of the treatment. A sharp blow to the lower sternum may cause ventricular fibrillation to revert spontaneously to sinus rhythm. If this does not occur, external cardiac massage should be commenced immediately using the heel of one hand placed on the lower half of the sternum with the other on top. Compressions to depress the sternum by 2 or 3 cm should be as slow as is compatible with achieving a rate of 80 compressions per minute. If ventilation is being controlled, one breath should be delivered for every four heart compressions. This method of cardiopulmonary resuscitation assumes that blood flow occurs because the heart is compressed between the sternum and the vertebral column.

An alternative hypothesis is that blood flow occurs because raised intrathoracic pressure during cardiac compression is transmitted to the carotid artery but not the jugular vein causing an arteriovenous pressure gradient. It has been suggested that simultaneous chest compression and ventilation at high pressures may be a more effective way to increase stroke volume and myocardial blood flow. The efficacy of this method has not been shown to be greater than traditional methods and may lead to a rise in intracranial pressure and a decrease in intracranial perfusion. It has not, therefore, been widely adopted.

When external cardiac massage and ventilation are in progress, an intravenous cannula should be inserted and the electrocardiogram can be monitored. When the rhythm is known, drug therapy can be commenced. Various drugs are used. A protocol for their use is suggested in Table 3.2.3. The first line drug for ventricular fibrillation is lignocaine in a

182

**Table 3.2.3 Protocol for cardiac arrest in adults**

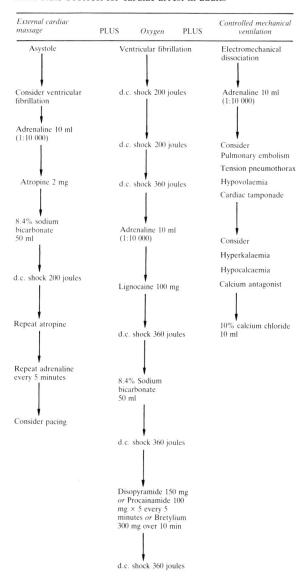

| _External cardiac massage_ | PLUS | _Oxygen_ | PLUS | _Controlled mechanical ventilation_ |
|---|---|---|---|---|
| Asystole | | Ventricular fibrillation | | Electromechanical dissociation |
| ↓ | | ↓ | | ↓ |
| Consider ventricular fibrillation | | d.c. shock 200 joules | | Adrenaline 10 ml (1:10 000) |
| ↓ | | ↓ | | ↓ |
| Adrenaline 10 ml (1:10 000) | | d.c. shock 200 joules | | Consider Pulmonary embolism Tension pneumothorax |
| ↓ | | ↓ | | Hypovolaemia Cardiac tamponade |
| Atropine 2 mg | | d.c. shock 360 joules | | |
| ↓ | | ↓ | | ↓ |
| 8.4% sodium bicarbonate 50 ml | | Adrenaline 10 ml (1:10 000) | | Consider Hyperkalaemia Hypocalcaemia |
| ↓ | | ↓ | | Calcium antagonist |
| d.c. shock 200 joules | | Lignocaine 100 mg | | |
| ↓ | | ↓ | | ↓ |
| Repeat atropine | | d.c. shock 360 joules | | 10% calcium chloride 10 ml |
| ↓ | | ↓ | | |
| Repeat adrenaline every 5 minutes | | 8.4% Sodium bicarbonate 50 ml | | |
| ↓ | | ↓ | | |
| Consider pacing | | d.c. shock 360 joules | | |
| | | ↓ | | |
| | | Disopyramide 150 mg _or_ Procainamide 100 mg × 5 every 5 minutes _or_ Bretylium 300 mg over 10 min | | |
| | | ↓ | | |
| | | d.c. shock 360 joules | | |

dose of 1 mg/kg body weight if defibrillation has failed to restore permanent sinus rhythm. If this fails and the fibrillation is fine, coarse ventricular fibrillation, which is more susceptible to successful defibrillation, may be induced by adrenaline. If ventricular fibrillation or ventricular dysrhythmias are persistent, procainamide or bretylium tosylate may be given. Sodium bicarbonate is also helpful if the arterial pH is less than 7.1. The formula is as follows:

volume of 8.4% sodium bicarbonate in ml

$$= \frac{0.3 \times \text{kg body weight} \times \text{base deficit}}{2}$$

Sodium bicarbonate can cause hypernatraemia, hyperosmality, paradoxical cerebral acidosis, myocardial depression and metabolic alkalosis with consequent tissue hypoxia. Where possible, arterial acid base status should be estimated prior to the administration of sodium bicarbonate.

The drug of first choice for asystole is adrenaline. This should only be given if the diagnosis of asystole is certain. It has been recommended that the patient should be defibrillated prior to the administration of adrenaline. This is because faulty equipment, the gain control turned down too low and fine ventricular fibrillation can cause ventricular fibrillation to be mistaken for asystole. If a sinus bradycardia or idioventricular bradycardia is present, it is often recommended that atropine should be given before adrenaline. If adrenaline does not restore sinus rhythm, sodium bicarbonate (after estimation of arterial acid base status), a repeat dose of adrenaline and then isoprenaline can be given. Ten per cent calcium chloride is also used if adrenaline does not reverse asystole but should be used with caution because it may increase mortality and excess cellular calcium influx may cause cerebral damage in the ischaemic brain.

Electromechanical dissociation is defined as a condition with normal electrocardiographic complexes without equivalent mechanical function of the heart. It can occur with cardiac tamponade or tension pneumothorax. Adrenaline, isoprenaline and calcium may improve myocardial function temporarily but resuscitation will not be successful unless the underlying cause is adequately treated.

It is customary to administer drugs by the intravenous route during cardiopulmonary resuscitation. In the absence of venous access, atropine, adrenaline and lignocaine can be administered by the tracheal route. The drugs are usually administered in 10–20 ml of physiological saline and dispersed by several hyperinflations of the lungs. Intratracheal absorption of these drugs is rapid in patients with a normal circulation and the effective doses are the same as the intravenous dose. During cardiac massage, the circulation is less than normal and higher doses are probably necessary. There is still some debate about the most effective doses for drugs administered by the intratracheal route during cardiac arrest, but the UK Resuscitation Council's recommendation that twice the intravenous dose should be given is widely accepted.

**Cardiac tamponade.** Fluid should be aspirated from the pericardial sac in the manner described for severely injured patients (p. 49).

**Tension pneumothorax.** The treatment is described on p. 49. Successful cardiopulmonary resuscitation is dependent on the recognition and treatment of the precipitating cause of the cardiac arrest.

**Myocardial failure.** If a normal cardiac rhythm can be obtained, it is likely that the failing myocardium will require inotropic assistance in order to maintain a normal cardiac output. The drug chosen will depend on associated factors such as the state of the vascular bed and the heart rate. The properties of commonly used inotropic agents are summarized in Table 3.2.4 but these effects are not always seen in every patient and the drug used should be tailored to each individual patient's response. In certain patients, a combination of drugs may produce the desired increase in cardiac output in lower doses than is achievable when either drug is used alone. Such a low dose combination may cause a lesser

**Table 3.2.4 Properties of cardiovascular drugs**

|                        | HR    | BP    | CO    | SVR                |
| ---------------------- | ----- | ----- | ----- | ------------------ |
| Adrenaline             | + +   | 0/+   | + +   | 0/+ +              |
| Noradrenaline          | +     | +     | +     | + +                |
| Isoprenaline           | + + + | +     | + + + | 0                  |
| Ephedrine              | +     | +     | +     | 0/+                |
| Dopamine               | 0/+   | 0/+   | +/+ + | −/+ (dose related) |
| Dobutamine             | 0/+   | 0/+   | + +   | 0/+                |
| Digoxin                | 0/−   | 0     | 0/+   | 0                  |
| Glucagon               | +     | +     | +     | −                  |
| Salbutamol             | +     | 0/−   | +     | −                  |
| Labetalol              | −     | −     | −     | −                  |
| Amrinone               | +     | 0/−   | + +   | −                  |
| ACE inhibitors         | −     | −     | + +   | − −                |
| Nitroglycerin          | +     | −     | −/+   | −                  |
| Sodium nitroprusside   | +     | −     | −/+   | −                  |
| Atropine               | + +   | 0/+   | +     | −                  |

increase in heart rate and less vasoconstriction than when either drug is used alone. Adrenaline and noradrenaline, when used alone, may increase cardiac output at the expense of inducing intense vasoconstriction and a reduction in renal blood flow but, if used in combination with a renal dose of dopamine, can increase cardiac output while renal function is maintained. Amiodarone is sometimes used for congestive cardiac failure but its vasodilator effects make it unsuitable for use in vasodilated, septic patients.

**Massive intracranial pathology**.   In patients in whom cardiac arrest is secondary to brain stem damage, cardiopulmonary resuscitation is unlikely to be successful. If, however, sinus rhythm is restored, the cardiac output is almost certain to be inadequate unless an inotrope such as dopamine is infused. Usually, cardiac arrest is one manifestation of actual or imminent brain stem death. Long-term survival in this group of patients is impossible if brain stem death has occurred or is in the process of occurring. The only justification for inotropic support is to maintain organ perfusion while formal brain stem death testing is carried out. This may be appropriate if the patient or his relatives have expressed the desire to donate organs for the purpose of transplantation.

### FURTHER READING

Opie, L.H. (1991). *Drugs for the Heart*, 3rd edn. Philadelphia: W.B. Saunders Co.
Chamberlain, D.A. (1989). Advanced life support. *Br. Med. J.*, **299**, 446–448.

# Difficulties in the management of cardiovascular insufficiency

The problems encountered in the medical and surgical patient are identical to those encountered in the severely injured patient. The reader is referred to pp. 51–54 for a detailed discussion of these problems and is reminded of the importance of monitoring the response to treatment in order to ensure that the response is appropriate to the treatment being given. An inadequate response implies either that treatment is insufficient or that the wrong diagnosis has been made. It is particularly important to distinguish between pump failure, hypovolaemia and non-circulatory causes of cardiovascular collapse such as tension pneumothorax or brain stem pathology.

# The causes and diagnosis of altered conscious level

A decrease in conscious level is a common cause for emergency admission to the A&E department. Transient loss of consciousness does not usually involve the anaesthetist. A prolonged alteration in consciousness may well involve the anaesthetist particularly if it is severe and is associated with inability to maintain the airway and an altered respiratory pattern. In an emergency the AVPU method (p. 59) can be used to describe the level of consciousness. A more detailed method of assessing conscious level is the Glasgow Coma Scale (p. 60) which was originally described for head injuries but is equally applicable to medical and surgical emergencies.

The causes of altered conscious level are numerous and are summarized in Table 3.2.5. A brief primary survey will

**Table 3.2.5 The causes of altered conscious level in adults**

| Intracranial pathological events | Head injury<br>Epilepsy<br>Tumour<br>Subdural/extradural haematoma | Cardiovascular accident<br>Subarachnoid haemorrhage<br>Hypertensive encephalopathy |
|---|---|---|
| Metabolic abnormalities | Primary hypoxia<br>Hypovolaemia (secondary hypoxia)<br>Hyperglycaemia<br>Hypoglycaemia<br>Hepatic coma<br>Myxoedema<br>Inappropriate ADH secretion | Hyperkalaemia<br>Hypernatraemia<br>Hyponatraemia<br>Dehydration<br>Water intoxication<br>Addisonian crisis<br>Uraemia |
| Poisoning (cerebral depression) | Opiates<br>Alcohol<br>Antidepressants<br>Anticonvulsants | Sedatives<br>Carbon monoxide<br>Cyanide<br>Solvents |
| Poisoning (fits) | Tricyclic antidepressants<br>Antihistamines | Phenothiazines<br><br>Theophyllines |
| Infective | Meningitis<br>Septicaemia | Encephalitis<br>Cerebral malaria |
| Miscellaneous | Hypothermia | Heat stroke |

reveal life-threatening deficiencies of the airway, breathing and circulation which may be due to the altered level of consciousness or may have caused it. The primary survey may also give clues to the diagnosis. Lacerations and boggy swellings of the scalp may indicate head injury, intracranial events may be indicated by obvious neurological deficits such as facial asymmetry or hemiplegia, injection marks may indicate drug abuse or diabetes and obvious abnormalities of body temperature may suggest heat stroke, infection or hypothermia as a cause of the unconsciousness. Once the airway, breathing and circulatory abnormalities have been treated, a secondary survey and investigations will help to make a definitive diagnosis. The doctor should obtain a detailed history from the ambulance staff, relatives or friends as a pre-existing medical condition which could precipitate the altered level of consciousness may be identified. The clinical examination should include a detailed neurological examination including the size and reactivity of the pupils. The doctor should also look for pyrexia, neck stiffness, signs of dehydration and the clinical stigmata of renal or hepatic disease. Investigations should include a full blood count, estimation of blood sugar and serum electrolytes and urea, a chest X-ray and other X-rays as indicated by the clinical findings. Blood should also be taken for toxicological testing if a drug overdose is suspected as the cause of the altered conscious level.

# Resuscitation and definitive management of altered conscious level

The anaesthetist's first concern should be to ensure that the airway is clear and, if airway reflexes are obtunded, protected by a cuffed endotracheal tube. Secondly, adequate ventilation and oxygenation must be guaranteed and, thirdly, cardiovascular insufficiency must be corrected. Some causes of life-threatening coma are rapidly remediable. Examples include gross hypoxia, severe hypovolaemia, hypoglycaemia and hyperglycaemia. If a rapid response to treatment is anticipated, the anaesthetist may consider maintaining the airway with manual methods. If this is not possible, intubation and ventilation are indicated. The use of muscle relaxants to facilitate intubation and ventilation may make subsequent neurological examination extremely difficult. If possible, a short-acting muscle relaxant should be used for endotracheal intubation and when it has worn off ventilation assisted manually without the administration of a longer acting muscle relaxant until the neurological examination is complete. At this stage a relatively short-acting muscle relaxant such as atracurium or vecuronium can be used. The advantage of these drugs is that they can be rapidly reversed to permit subsequent neurological assessments. Many anaesthetists favour vecuronium because of the low incidence of allergic reactions it causes. Atracurium may, however, be preferable if the diagnosis has not been clearly established as it undergoes Hoffman degradation at body temperature and pH and does not depend on renal or hepatic function for its elimination.

If the patient has ingested an overdose of drugs, the anaesthetist may be called upon to protect the airway while a gastric lavage is performed. It is particularly important to avoid the pulmonary inhalation of gastric contents during endotracheal intubation. It is also important to use short acting drugs which will not affect subsequent assessment of the patient. Drugs should only be used if they are absolutely necessary. If the patient is not deeply unconscious, propofol is a suitable agent to produce unconsciousness. Suxamethonium is the agent of choice to produce muscle relaxation.

Certain drugs cause cardiac dysrhythmias. These can be treated by the methods described on pp. 192–194. The definitive treatment of unconsciousness from other causes is not usually indicated in the A&E department.

# Monitoring life-saving resuscitation and the response to definitive treatment

Monitoring during the resuscitation period will be similar to that described for the severely injured patient (pp. 54–63). Initially, simple, non-invasive measures are appropriate. These can be supplanted by more invasive techniques as life-saving measures become effective and definitive treatment is begun.

Specific mention should be made of the value of a full blood count, urea and electolyte and blood sugar estimation in medical and surgical patients. These monitoring parameters are far more likely to produce useful information in medical and surgical emergency patients than they are in severely injured patients. There are several reasons for this. First, the patient population is far older and therefore more likely to suffer from diseases such as diabetes, renal impairment or to be on medication such as diuretics which may cause electrolyte abnormalities. Second, diseases such as chronic bronchitis and cancer can ultimately cause an emergency admission but are insidious in onset, and may cause significant alterations in the full blood count such as polycythaemia or anaemia. Finally, prolonged bowel obstruction causing diarrhoea and vomiting will significantly alter serum electrolytes and inflammatory or infective diseases may increase the white cell count. These are but a few examples of the abnormalities which may be anticipated in medical and surgical patients and which may assist with the diagnosis or require correction as part of the treatment plan.

# Specific diseases of importance to the anaesthetist

## *Cardiac dysrhythmias*

Life-threatening dysrhythmias which have significance for the resuscitation of severely ill and injured persons are those which compromise cardiac output. Several mechanisms account for the reduction in cardiac output caused by dysrhythmias. In general, urgent treatment of a dysrhythmia is indicated if the systolic blood pressure is less than 90 mmHg, if the peripheral circulation is constricted, if there is an alteration in conscious level or if the dysrhythmia has caused myocardial failure and pulmonary oedema.

**The pathophysiological causes of reduced cardiac output**. Cardiac output depends on the ventricular rate and is maximal at ventricular rates of 80 to 100 beats per minute. Although ventricular filling is the most important factor influencing cardiac output, atrial activity is also relevant. Diastolic filling is mostly passive and depends on the pressure gradient between the atria and ventricles. In the last third of diastole, however, atrial contraction contibutes to the total stroke volume. The atrial contribution to stroke volume is important at higher heart rates and in patients with ventricular insufficiency. Patients in whom the atria do not contract or in whom the atria contract in the wrong part of the cardiac cycle are more prone to hypotension. At heart rates below 40 beats per minute, cardiac output may fall significantly although young fit athletes may normally have rates at this level which are compensated for by an increase in ventricular contractility. At heart rates above 120 beats per minute, the time available for ventricular filling is reduced to the extent that cardiac output begins to fall and at rates above 160 beats per minute the fall in cardiac output becomes clinically significant. These values apply to patients with normal atrial function. If the end diastolic atrial contribution to cardiac output is absent, clinically significant falls in cardiac output may occur at rates as low as 130 beats per minute. These figures should only be used as guidelines for initiating treatment. The clinical response should be used only as a guide because the ability of the patient to compensate for falls in cardiac output will also depend on factors such as the adequacy of vascular filling, the ability of the vessels to constrict and the adequacy of myocardial contractility.

**Atrial fibrillation or flutter**.   It is unusual for these dysrhythmias to cause a life-threatening reduction in cardiac output. If they do, sinus rhythm may be restored by a 50 joule d.c. countershock or by rapid intravenous digitalization with 0.75–1 mg digoxin.

**Supraventricular tachycardia**.   Carotid sinus massage may restore sinus rhythm but if it fails a 50 joule synchronized d.c. shock is the treatment of choice.

193

**Sinus bradycardia**. Intravenous atropine 0.6–1.2 mg is usually successful. If this fails isoprenaline given as an infusion at a dose of 10 μg/min will increase the heart rate. Bradycardia due to excessive beta blockade is particularly resistant to treatment. In addition to atropine and isoprenaline, it may be necessary to give an infusion of dobutamine starting at a dose of 10 μg/kg/min or a bolus dose of 50 μg/kg glucagon followed by an infusion given at a rate of 1–5 mg/hour to increase the cardiac output. If drug therapy fails or is only temporarily successful, cardiac pacing may be required.

**Ventricular tachycardia**. If the blood pressure is low, the treatment of choice is a synchronized 200 joule d.c. countershock. If the blood pressure is maintained, intravenous lignocaine in a dose of 1 mg/kg body weight can be used. If lignocaine does not cause a reversion to sinus rhythm, intravenous procainamide 200 mg or synchronized d.c. countershock may be used.

**Ventricular fibrillation**. The treatment of ventricular fibrillation is described on p. 184.

**FURTHER READING**

Opie, L.H. (1991). *Drugs for the Heart*, 3rd edn. Philadelphia: W.B. Saunders Co.

# *Septicaemia*

Septicaemia should be suspected if a patient is admitted to the A&E department with unexplained hypotension, oliguria or a confusional state associated with a raised or lowered body temperature. The original site of infection may be the lungs or heart valves, abdomen, central nervous system or in the soft tissues or joints. Common pathogens are *Escherichia coli, Staphylococcus aureus, Staphylococcus epidermidis* and *Streptococcus pneumoniae*.

**Pathophysiological changes**. The pathophysiological response in septicaemia is similar no matter what the infecting organism or the original site of infection and appears to be based on the release from monocytes of Interleukin–1 and tumour necrosis factor, in response to circulating endotoxins from the infecting organism. These toxins are just two of a number of toxins which are thought to be involved in the clinical spectrum of features which characterize septicaemia. Histamine, beta endorphins, components of the complement cascade and arachidonic acid metabolites have all been implicated in the vasodilatation and decreased systemic vascular resistance which causes relative hypovolaemia in septic patients. Vasoactive amines, endotoxin itself and angiotensin, with or without hypoxaemia and a metabolic acidosis, have been blamed for the pulmonary hypertension which is a common feature of septicaemia. In addition to relative hypovolaemia, septic patients also have absolute hypovolaemia due to the leak of serum from capillaries. Again, several mediators which cause increased capillary permeability have been identified. They include tumour necrosis factor, superoxides, proteases and leukotrienes. Biventricular myocardial failure is also common in sepsis and is probably due to hypoxia, diminished coronary blood flow, toxins and abnormal calcium flux within myocardial cells. Oxygen flux in the tissues is frequently abnormal in septic patients and oxygen consumption is delivery dependent. This may be due to shunting and maldistribution of blood flow within the tissues or due to an inability of the cells to utilize oxygen normally.

**Management of septicaemia**. The clinical presentation of septic shock is variable. Classically the patient is febrile, tachypnoeic, hypotensive, peripherally vasodilated and has a hyperdynamic circulation. The diagnosis of septicaemia in this group of patients must be differentiated from acute pancreatitis and hepatic failure. If the septicaemia is relatively long standing, the patient may be hypotensive and peripherally vasoconstricted with a poor urine output, in which case cardiogenic shock, pulmonary embolism and hypovolaemia must be ruled out as possible diagnoses.

In the A&E department, the treatment of septic shock is usually limited to life-saving measures. The airway should be secured, adequate ventilation and oxygenation ensured and cardiovascular insufficiency treated. During life-saving resuscitation, repeated challenges with 200 ml of a colloidal solution should be given until there is no further rise in blood pressure. If hypotension is unresponsive to colloids, inotropic support should be considered. If the patient has warm peripheries, noradrenaline as an infusion given at a rate of 2–10 µg/min is a suitable choice because it will constrict the peripheral vasculature as well as providing inotropic support.

If the patient has vasoconstricted peripheries, dopamine given as an infusion at a rate of up to 20 µg/kg/min is probably a better inotrope to start with. If inotropic support is required, it will be necessary to use a pulmonary artery flotation catheter to monitor subsequent treatment. It is arguable whether the A&E department is the ideal place to commence this type of monitoring. A temporary central venous pressure catheter may be more suitable, but as soon as the patient has been stabilized rapid transfer to the Intensive Care Unit should be considered. Whatever the relative merits of the central venous pressure catheter as opposed to the pulmonary artery flotation catheter for monitoring, it is essential that vasoactive drugs are given through a central vein as extravasation from a cannula in a peripheral vein can cause intense local vasoconstriction and skin loss.

# Poisoning

Poisoning can occur with a huge variety of substances and may be accidental or self inflicted. Certain poisonous agents such as iron or paracetamol may be life threatening in the long term but have relatively innocuous immediate effects. The discussion in this section does not include late life-threatening effects of poisons and is confined to immediate life-threatening problems encountered in the A&E department. Although it is not essential to know which poison is involved in order to initiate life-saving measures, a history from relatives or the ambulance staff is helpful because knowledge of the poison will enable the doctor to anticipate potential problems.

**Life-threatening pathophysiological effects of poisoning**. Poisons may induce hypoxia directly as occurs in carbon monoxide or cyanide poisoning or indirectly by causing coma and airway obstruction, convulsions, pulmonary aspiration of vomit, respiratory depression or a combination of these problems. Cardiovascular insufficiency may be caused by dysrhythmias, reduction of myocardial contractility or vaso-dilatation. These life-threatening problems are induced by a variety of drugs (Table 3.3.1).

**Management**.   The anaesthetist's attention should be directed to administering oxygen and securing the airway. This is usually easy although, if corrosive substances have been ingested, laryngeal damage and swelling is a potential problem which should be anticipated and prepared for (pp. 132–133). Secondly, adequate ventilation must be established. Finally, circulatory insufficiency must be dealt with. Dysrhythmias should be treated as described on pp. 192–194. Hypovolaemia is not usually severe and will respond to elevation of the foot of the bed and transfusion of a crystalloid solution. If these measures fail, myocardial depression may be a contributory cause of circulatory insufficiency and the use of a dobutamine or dopamine infusion should be considered.

Definitive management such as gastric lavage (except if corrosive agents have been ingested ) and the administration of specific antidotes should be carried out when life-saving resuscitative measures have been commenced. The anaes-

**Table 3.3.1 Life-threatening effects of poisoning**

| | |
|---|---|
| Coma | Tricyclic antidepressants<br>Opiates<br>Sedatives<br>Anti-epileptic medication<br>Alcohol<br>Lithium<br>Carbon monoxide<br>Cyanide<br>Salicylates<br>Organophosphate insecticides |
| Dysrhythmias | Tricyclic antidepressants<br>Drugs for control of cardiac rhythm,<br>hypertension and angina<br>Theophyllines |
| Hypotension | Drugs for dysrhythmias and hypertension<br>Paraquat<br>Cyanide<br>Opiates<br>Sedatives |
| Respiratory depression | Opiates<br>Sedatives<br>Alcohol<br>Carbon monoxide<br>Cyanide<br>Tricyclic antidepressants |
| Pulmonary oedema | Paraquat<br>Salicylates<br>Hydrocarbons and petroleum products, e.g.<br>white spirit, polish, window cleaners<br>Organophosphate insecticides |
| Hypoglycaemia | Insulin<br>Oral hypoglycaemics<br>Salicylates<br>Alcohol |

thetist is not usually required to administer the antidotes but a knowledge of those available is helpful as the prompt administration of an antidote such as naloxone or flumazenil may obviate the need for endotracheal intubation and ventilation. The antidotes which may be useful are listed in Table 3.3.2.

# Cardiogenic shock and myocardial failure

Cardiogenic shock is generally due to a large myocardial infarction. Less commonly it may be due to a smaller infarction in a patient who has had several previous infarctions, traumatic myocardial contusion, carbon monoxide and cyanide poisoning, septal perforation, acute valvular insuffi-

**Table 3.3.2 Specific antidotes to poisons**

| Poison | Antidote |
| --- | --- |
| Opiate | Naloxone up to 1.2 mg IV |
| Benzodiazepine | Flumazenil 200 μg IV followed by 100 μg boluses at 1-minute intervals up to a total dose of 1 mg |
| Beta blockers | Glucagon 5 mg IV |
| Cyanide | Dicobalt edetate 600 mg IV or 30% sodium nitrite 10 ml *plus* 50% sodium thiosulphate 50 ml over 10 minutes |
| Carbon monoxide | 100% of hyperbaric oxygen |
| Organophosphate insecticides | Atropine 2 mg *and* Pralidoxime 1 g in 250 ml physiological saline over 1 hour |

ciency, an atrial myoxoma, cardiomyopathy or myocarditis. The clinical features of cardiogenic shock include a reduction in systolic blood pressure of at least 30 mmHg, mental confusion, peripheral vasoconstriction and oliguria or anuria. Pulmonary oedema secondary to myocardial failure may occur. Other features of myocardial infarction such as acute chest pain and dysrhythmias may also be present.

**Pathophysiology of cardiogenic shock.**   Cardiogenic shock occurs if there is a reduction in ventricular function of more than 40%. This usually reduces the cardiac index to less than 2 l/min/ m$^2$ . Failure of the heart to pump effectively induces an intense neurohumoral response which increases the heart rate and causes massive vasoconstriction. This is usually insufficient to compensate for the reduction in myocardial function and causes generalized tissue hypoxia. As with severely injured, burned or septic patients, cellular dysfunction and death from hypoxia can result in multiple organ failure. In the patient with cardiogenic shock, multiple organ failure is rarely a problem as the mortality rate from the initial episode is high unless there is a surgically remediable lesion.

**Management of cardiogenic shock.**   Life-saving measures begin with the administration of oxygen. If this does not correct hypoxia or there is airway or respiratory insufficiency, endotracheal intubation and ventilation are indicated. Sedative drugs and muscle relaxants should be chosen with care (Table 1.3.5, p. 84) as they may cause vasodilatation or myocardial depression and aggravate hypotension. Similarly, the rise in intrathoracic pressure caused by controlled mechanical ventilation may reduce venous return and induce hypotension. A ventilatory pattern which produces adequate oxygenation with the least rise in intrathoracic pressure should be chosen. Severe pulmonary oedema impairs oxygenation and may respond to the use of positive end expiratory pressure in addition to diuretics and aminophylline. Inevitably, the use of positive end expiratory pressure increases intrathoracic pressure. An improvement in oxygenation may be achieved at the expense of a further reduction in cardiac index. Inotropic agents such as dopamine or dobutamine may also be required. The improvement in myocardial contractility may, however, be achieved at the expense of increased myocardial oxygen consumption and, if this cannot be matched by increased coronary blood flow and oxygen delivery, further areas of myocardial muscle may be put at risk.

When an improvement in systemic blood pressure has been achieved, a further improvement in myocardial efficiency may occur if vasodilators such as sodium nitroprusside, nitroglycerin, salbutamol or ACE inhibitors are given. These agents reduce myocardial work by reducing systemic vascular resistance, causing pooling of the blood in the venous circulation and a reduction in the severity of pulmonary oedema and possibly improved flow of blood to the tissues, hence reducing tissue hypoxia. The intra-aortic balloon pump has also been used to assist the failing myocardium.

The extent of treatment in the A&E department is debatable. It should probably be limited to basic measures such as intubation, ventilation, the use of an inotropic infusion and emergency treatment of dysrhythmias. Subsequent changes in inotropic agents, the administration of vasodilators and the use of the intra-aortic balloon pump require monitoring with a pulmonary artery flotation catheter and are best carried out in the Coronary or Intensive Care Unit.

# *Pulmonary embolism*

In the A&E department, the anaesthetist will probably be called only to patients who have suffered a massive pulmonary embolism. The patient will give a history of recent immobility because of prolonged travel or hospital admission or may have been on the contraceptive pill and will be complaining of severe breathlessness, haemoptysis, pleuritic chest pain and faintness due to hypotension. The patient will be cyanosed. In the presence of a massive pulmonary embolism, the chest X-ray may appear normal or show oligaemia. The electrocardiogram may be normal or show right axis deviation, right bundle branch block, sinus tachycardia, and an inverted T wave and Q wave in lead III. Atrial flutter of fibrillation may also be seen.

**Pathophysiological changes due to pulmonary embolism**.  A massive pulmonary embolism often affects both pulmonary arteries. Blood flow through the lungs is dramatically reduced, not only by the mechanical effects of the embolus but also by a vasoconstrictive response of the pulmonary vasculature. Although there is a reduction in alveolar ventilation, this response is inefficient in comparison to reflex pulmonary, hypoxic vasoconstriction and thus there is a significant imbalance between ventilation and perfusion which means that pulmonary embolism can cause severe hypoxia. Hypercarbia is not usually a problem as carbon dioxide clearance is achieved by increased ventilation of the unaffected parts of the lung.

Cardiac output does not usually fall until 50% of the pulmonary circulation has been obstructed by an embolus, at which stage pulmonary artery pressure increases. The increase in pulmonary artery pressure causes right ventricular failure and tricuspid incompetence. Cardiac output may be further reduced by concomitant atrial fibrillation or flutter. Indeed, it may have been the onset of a dysrhythmia that dislodged a mural thrombus which had developed in a diseased heart and caused the pulmonary embolism. The result of suboptimal oxygenation of the bood and reduced blood flow to the tissues is tissue hypoxia.

**Management of pulmonary embolism**.  The primary problem is reduced blood flow through the lungs and to the heart. Oxygen will increase the amount of available oxygen in the lungs which can be transferred to the blood. Controlled mechanical ventilation does not usually improve oxygenation of the blood as the alveoli are initially uninvolved in the disease process. Furthermore, controlled mechanical ventilation may reduce venous return and hence further compromise the cardiac output. Treatment is designed to improve pulmonary perfusion and blood flow to the heart. A colloid infusion will increase right ventricular filling pressures and may improve blood flow to the heart. Rapid digitalization will improve myocardial function in the presence of atrial flutter or fibrillation. If, in spite of these measures, hypotension persists, the cardiac output can be increased by an infusion of dobutamine or noradrenaline. A heparin infusion can be started to prevent extension of the clot. All of these measures can be commenced in the A&E department. Ultimately, however, clinical improvement can only be obtained by removal of the clot. This will occur slowly by inherent lytic processes. The rapidity of clinical improvemant can be enhanced by the administration of streptokinase or by surgical removal of the clot. Neither of these treatment options should be considered without radiological assessment of the extent and location of the embolism. Nor is the A&E department an appropriate place for this type of therapy.

# *Asthma*

Patients with an acute attack of severe asthma present to the A&E department with acute breathlessness. There is usually a history of poor control during the preceding weeks or the acute onset of a respiratory tract infection. The anaesthetist may be asked to assist with the management of patients with severe asthma who are in imminent need of controlled mechanical ventilation. The patient will be extremely breathless and unable to talk without frequent pauses. He will be breathing rapidly and using the accessory muscles of respiration. He may be confused or agitated due to cerebral hypoxia. If the patient is capable of using a peak flow metre, a peak expiratory flow rate of less than 150 l/min indicates a severe attack. The pulse rate will be rapid. This could be solely due to anxiety, but more probably reflects the increased work of breathing or the use of sympathomimetic drugs. Pulsus paradoxus due to the increased negative intra-thoracic pressure will be evident. The systolic blood pressure may be reduced. On examination, overinflation of the chest will be evident and musical rhonchi will be heard all over the chest. In extremely severe cases, the rhonchi may be very soft because airflow is so severely restricted that turbulence is minimal.

**Pathophysiological changes due to asthma**.   The airways of asthmatic patients contain hypertrophied smooth muscle, oedematous mucosa and hypertrophied mucous glands. These glands produce thick tenacious mucus which forms plugs which obstruct the airways. An acute attack of asthma is thought to be initiated by an antigen–antibody reaction which stimulates the release of mediators such as histamine, prostaglandins and bradykinins which cause a reduction in intracellular cyclic-AMP and hence smooth muscle contraction. Capillary permeability is increased by these mediators and receptors in the bronchial wall are stimulated and activate the vagus nerve, inducing bronchoconstriction. During an attack of asthma, expiratory gas flow is reduced. The abnormality in ventilation and mucus plugging of the airways causes an inequality between ventilation and perfusion which cannot be completely corrected by hypoxic pulmonary vaso-constriction. Hence, asthmatics are hypoxic. Hyperventilation maintains normocarbia until the patient becomes exhausted when hypercarbia becomes evident. Hypercarbia is, therefore, an ominous sign as it usually means that controlled mechanical ventilation is required.

**Management of severe asthma**.   The patient should be sat up and given oxygen through a face mask. If possible the oxygen should be humidified as this may help to loosen thick mucus secretions. If there is time, bronchodilators should be given. These are administered by various routes and fall into three chemical groups. The first group contains beta 2-adrenergic agonists which increase adenyl cyclase activity and hence the intracellular concentration of cyclic-AMP. Drugs in this group include salbutamol, ephedrine and terbutaline. The second group of drugs are the methylxanthines which increase the concentration of cyclic-AMP by inhibiting phosphodiesterase. Aminophylline and theophylline are examples of this type of drug. At toxic levels (serum theophylline greater than 40 mg/l) life-threatening dysrhythmias and convulsions may occur. These drugs should, therefore, be given with caution and ideally serum theophylline levels should be measured as soon as possible. The third group of drugs are the parasympatholytic agents which inhibit vagal activity. Many of these drugs have a systemic atropine-like effect and cause tachycardia, inhibition of ciliary activity and drying of secretions. Ipratropium bromide does not have systemic effects and is the most commonly used drug in this group. Although its bronchodilator action is weak, it has a synergistic effect with beta 2-agonists. Steroids are also given to severe cases but their onset of action is slow and the mechanism of their effect is not clearly understood. Suggested dosages for drugs used in the treatment of acute asthma are given in Table 3.2.2, on p. 178.

Many patients are dehydrated and are unable to take oral fluids. An intravenous infusion of crystalloid solution is indicated for rehydration although overload should be avoided as capillary permeability is increased and mucosal oedema may be worsened.

If these measures are insufficient, controlled mechanical ventilation is indicated. There is, however, a significant risk that mechanical ventilation will result in air trapping and hyperinflation of the lungs which may result in barotrauma or hypotension. The severity of hyperinflation depends on the tidal volume, expiratory time and the severity of airflow obstruction. The ventilator must be carefully adjusted to minimize hyperinflation. Small tidal volumes given at a relatively rapid rate are usually most effective. The inspiratory flow should be as rapid as possible in order to allow the longest possible period for expiration. The minute volume should be the minimum required to oxygenate the patient and to maintain arterial carbon dioxide level so that the arterial pH is greater than 7.2. This will minimize the risk of barotrauma and hypotension. As the degree of airway obstruction decreases the ventilator can be repeatedly adjusted to improve carbon dioxide clearance.

In order to ventilate the patient, endotracheal intubation will be required and anaesthesia or sedation will be required. Ketamine, halothane and ether are bronchodilators and it is worth considering their use for the purposes of anaesthesia prior to intubation.

# *Meningitis*

The classical signs of meningitis include fever, headache, neck stiffness, vomiting, photophobia, coma, fits and cranial nerve palsies. A purpuric rash is common in meningococcal septicaemia. Most of these cases are managed by physicians. Sometimes, however, meningitis causes coma, seizures or septic shock. The septic shock associated with meningococcal meningitis is notorious for the rapidity with which it can cause death. The anaesthetist's role is likely to be confined to the management of the effects of unconsciousness and septic shock. The pathophysiological problems of unconsciousness and their management have been described on pp. 187–190. The pathophysiological changes of septic shock have all the features described on pp. 194–195 and the management is similar (pp. 195–196). The anaesthetist should be aware that bilateral adrenal haemorrhage is a complication of meningococcal septicaemia and may contribute to hypotension. It responds to 300 mg of hydrocortisone given intravenously.

# Guillain–Barré syndrome

The Guillain Barré syndrome frequently follows a minor viral illness. Its onset is characterized by the development of paraesthesiae in the hands and feet followed by the development of motor weakness in the limbs. Severe cases may develop paralysis of the cranial and intercostal nerves.

**The pathophysiological changes of Guillain–Barré syndrome.** The syndrome is thought to be due to immunological nerve injury. Peripheral, autonomic and cranial nerves may be affected. In addition to the sensory and motor changes already mentioned which may result in respiratory failure and loss of protective airway reflexes, abnormalities of the autonomic nervous system may cause hypotension, bradycardia or paroxysmal tachycardias which are severe enough to cause cardiovascular insufficiency and paroxysmal hypertension which can cause myocardial failure or intracerebral haemorrhage. Furthermore, the response to some drugs is exaggerated. These drugs include nitroglycerin, ephedrine, dopamine, isoprenaline, thiopentone, morphine and frusemide. Suxamethonium may cause dysrhythmias or cardiac arrest secondary to hyperkalaemia. The mechanism is probably related to abnormalities of the muscle cell membrane.

**Management of the Guillain–Barré syndrome.** In the A&E department, it is unlikely that the syndrome will have progressed far enough to require the presence of an anaesthetist. Very rarely, the anaesthetist may be confronted with a patient who has obtunded airway reflexes or who has respiratory failure. The treatment consists of endotracheal intubation to protect the airway and mechanical ventilation. The drugs used to facilitate intubation and ventilation should be chosen with caution in order to avoid life-threatening alterations in pulse rate and blood pressure. If there is persistent hypotension which is severe enough to compromise renal and cerebral perfusion, transfusion of colloids and the cautious use of inotropic drugs is indicated. Hypertension can be treated by small incremental doses or an infusion of labetalol. Bradycardia may be resistant to atropine and require temporary pacing.

# *Status epilepticus*

Status epilepticus is defined as repeated fits occurring with such frequency that recovery between fits does not occur or continuous seizure activity lasting more than 30 minutes. The condition may occur in poorly controlled epileptics or be due to a variety of other causes such as a cerebral tumour, cerebrovascular accident, intracranial infection, gross cerebral hypoxia, drugs including tricyclic antidepressants, theophylline and cocaine, alcohol, benzodiazepine or narcotic withdrawal, electrolyte disturbances or hypoglycaemia.

**Pathophysiology of status epilepticus**. Prolonged seizures place unbearable demands on cerebral metabolic processes and may deplete cerebral nutrient stores. Permanent cell damage, cerebral oedema and lactic acid production occur. This damage can be compounded by hypoxic damage due to loss of airway control and respiratory depression secondary to the convulsion or to an overdose of anti-epileptic medication such as diazepam or thiopentone. In addition, cerebral hypoxia and cell damage may be worsened by hypotension which is a side effect of large doses of phenytoin

**Management of status epilepticus**. Initially, airway, breathing and circulatory insufficiency must be recognized and treated. Oxygen should be given to all patients, the airway secured, if necessary by endotracheal intubation and adequate ventilation established. Hypotension usually responds to an infusion of crystalloid solution. Having initiated life-saving resuscitation, the fits may be controlled in a variety of

**Table 3.3.3 The control of convulsions in adults**

| First | Diazepam up to 20 mg IV *or* paraldehyde 5 ml deep IM into each buttock |
| | Phenytoin 50 mg/min IV up to 1000 mg |
| If no response | 0.8% Chloromethiazole infusion rapidly until fitting stops |
| | Thiopentone 25–100 mg IV slowly |
| Still no response | Thiopentone 250 mg IV *plus* suxamethonium 100 mg IV |
| Plus | Controlled mechanical ventilation |

ways (Table 3.3.3). An attempt should be made to identify precipitating causes of the convulsion. In the A&E department, it is vital to test the blood sugar and to treat hypoglycaemia.

# *Diabetes mellitus*

Diabetics may be admitted to the A&E department in a coma due to either hypoglycaemia or hyperglycaemia. The diagnosis may be inferred from the history given by ambulance staff or relatives and confirmed by the measurement of blood sugar. Abnormalities in blood sugar level may be due to poor control of the disease or be precipitated in a previously well controlled diabetic by stress due to injury or severe disease. Sepsis is commonly accompanied by hyperglycaemia.

Unconsciousness may cause loss of airway control or loss of protective airway reflexes. Usually, prompt commencement of treatment to restore the blood sugar to normal levels is sufficient to restore normal upper airway function. In the interim, the administration of oxygen, use of the left lateral

209

**Table 3.3.4 The emergency management of hyperglycaemia in adults**

| | | |
|---|---|---|
| Start intravenous infusion | | |
| Physiological saline 1 l/hour for 2 hours, then 1 l over 2 hours | | |
| | | |
| Give soluble insulin | | |
| Soluble insulin | 10 i.u. IV stat, then 4–6 i.u./hour by infusion | |
| | *or* | |
| | 20 i.u. IM stat, then 10 i.u. every hour | |
| | | |
| Check serum potassium | | |
| Serum potassium | 3–6 mmol/l | 20 mmol KCl/hour |
| | <3 mmol/l | 40 mmol/KCl/hour |
| | >6 mmol/l | no KCl |

position and drainage of the stomach contents through a nasogastic tube is sufficient to ensure the patient's safety. Rarely, endotracheal intubation may be required. The treatment of abnormal blood sugar levels is usually managed by the physicians. A brief summary is given in Table 3.3.4. Hypotension can be a problem. It usually responds to an infusion of crystalloid solution but this should not be given as an isolated treatment modality. It should form part of the regime being used to control blood sugar.

# *Anaphylaxis*

Anaphylaxis is an immediate hypersensitivity reaction mediated in a previously sensitized individual by IgE antibody. Such reactions may be produced by snake and insect stings, foods and vaccines. Anaphylactoid reactions are clinically indistinguishable from anaphylactic reactions but are not antibody mediated and there may be no history of previous exposure to the precipitating agent. The clinical features may include generalized reddening of the skin, urticaria, angio-oedema which may be life threatening if it involves the larynx or respiratory tract, tachycardia, hypotension, bronchospasm and pulmonary oedema. Not all the clinical features occur with equal frequency. Cardiovascular changes and flushes occur in the majority of patients. Bronchospasm occurs in 40% and cardiac arrest in about 15% of patients. The speed of onset varies from a few seconds to 30 minutes from exposure to the precipitating agent. Death is usually due to laryngeal obstruction, severe bronchospasm or circulatory failure.

**Pathophysiological changes of anaphylactic and anaphylactoid reactions**. Anaphylactic reactions are initiated by the antigen-IgE antibody complex. Mast cell degranulation occurs and histamine and other mediators are released. These cause vasodilatation, increased capillary permeability and constriction of bronchiolar smooth muscle. During anaphylactoid reactions, similar changes are observed and are probably due to activation of the complement cascade and histamine release. The effects of these changes are to produce hypoxia and circulatory insufficiency which together cause severe tissue hypoxia.

**Management of anaphylactic and anaphylactoid reactions**. Oxygen should be given and, if necessary, the airway secured by endotracheal intubation and ventilation established. The problems of intubation in the presence of laryngeal oedema are similar to those encountered in burned patients (pp. 132–133) and the problems of treating a patient with severe bronchospasm are similar to those for treating an asthmatic (pp. 204–206). Hypotension is a reflection of relative hypovolaemia secondary to vasodilatation and absolute hypovolaemia due to fluid loss through leaking capillaries. Large volumes of colloidal solutions may be required to restore the blood pressure. Sometimes the vasodilatation is so extreme that the patient has impalpable pulses. External cardiac massage is indicated in this situation as it is in the case of true cardiac arrest.

Following basic measures to maintain the adequacy of airway, breathing and circulation, adrenaline 0.5 mg intravenously or through the endotracheal tube is very helpful. It increases myocardial contractility, causes vasoconstriction and relaxes bronchial smooth muscle.

If adrenaline does not relieve bronchospasm, an infusion of aminophylline may be helpful.

# Acute upper gastrointestinal haemorrhage

Acute upper gastrointestinal haemorrhage has many causes and is most commonly due to erosion of a gastric or duodenal ulcer. These patients may become severely hypotensive and have reduced levels of consciousness. They react to bleeding in exactly the same way as injured patients and the pathophysiological changes leading to tissue hypoxia are the same. Life-saving resuscitation is the same and if blood loss continues definitive surgical management is required to control it. The reader is referred to pp. 48–49 for further information.

Rarely, acute gastrointestinal haemorrhage is due to bleeding oesophageal varices. In this situation definitive management may include placement of a Sengstaken–Blakemore tube to tamponade the varices or the administration of vasopressin 24 units over 15 minutes and then 24 units per hour thereafter and nitroglycerin 2 mg/hour initially, increasing over the next two hours to 10 mg/hour. Both reduce portal pressure and hence bleeding.

# Ruptured aortic aneurysm, ruptured ectopic pregnancy and other causes of intra-abdominal haemorrhage

All causes of intra-abdominal bleeding may result in hypovolaemic shock and tissue hypoxia. As in the event of major upper gastrointestinal bleeding or bleeding from major injuries, the patient should be rapidly assessed and treated for airway, breathing and circulatory insufficiency. Blood loss must be replaced as rapidly and accurately as possible (pp. 48–49). Definitive surgical management is ultimately required to stop the bleeding. Usually, however, there is time for the anaesthetist to restore the circulating blood volume to normal before anaesthesia is induced and surgery commenced. If the bleeding is torrential, it may be necessary for surgery and resuscitation to proceed concurrently.

# Hypothermia

Hypothermia is usually defined as a core temperature of less than 35°C. The elderly and very young are at greater risk than other age groups because temperature control at the extremes of age is less effective. Hypothermia may be caused by immersion or exposure in otherwise healthy individuals. Frequently, however, it is associated with some other disease which renders the patient less able to take active measures to keep warm. Mild hypothermia is relatively common amongst patients admitted as emergencies to the A&E department. The anaesthetist does not usually become involved until the body temperature has fallen to below 32°C, at which temperature, life-threatening pathophysiological changes begin to occur.

**Pathophysiological changes of hypothermia**. At temperatures of less than 32°C, the heart rate, cardiac output and blood pressure begin to fall. Dysrhythmias such as atrial fibrillation may occur and the respiratory rate falls. The patient is apathetic and confused. Shivering has been replaced by muscle rigidity.

At 28°C, ventricular fibrillation is a significant risk but it may occur at higher temperatures in response to noxious stimuli such as endotracheal intubation or if the myocardium is diseased. The respiratory rate falls further and the minute volume lessens. Protective airway reflexes become obtunded. The oxygen dissociation curve shifts to the left, increasing the affinity of haemoglobin for oxygen. As respiratory depression worsens, however, a respiratory acidosis develops. Blood viscosity increases and tissue blood flow decreases causing tissue hypoxia and lactate production and hence a metabolic acidosis. Muscle weakness and eventually paralysis develop. The patient is comatose. Initially the blood glucose is increased due partly to decreased insulin release and partly to impaired peripheral utilization of glucose. The basal metabolic rate falls but eventually, as glycogen stores become depleted, hypoglycaemia may develop. Renal function and intestinal mobility are also decreased. Electrolyte abnormalities are common but unpredictable in their nature. At 26°C, the patient becomes areflexic and at 25°C respiration is completely inhibited. Death should never be assumed until the patient has been rewarmed to a body temperature of at least 28°C and resuscitation attempts have failed.

**Management of hypothermia**. Oxygen should be given, the airway protected and, if necessary, ventilation commenced. All manoeuvres should be performed as gently as possible to avoid precipitating ventricular fibrillation. If possible inspired gases should be warmed and humidified. Intravenous access should be secured so that warmed fluids can be given. They should be administered cautiously as pulmonary oedema may occur during rewarming if excessive amounts have been transfused. At low temperatures, ventricular fibrillation is resistant to treatment and prolonged external cardiac massage may be necessary until the body temperature has risen above 28°C. Bradycardia may also be resistant to atropine at low temperatures and may have to be treated by pacing. Intravenous glucose and sodium bicarbonate should be given for hypoglycaemia and acidosis respectively. Electrolyte abnormalities normally correct themselves as the body temperature increases.

Passive rewarming by placing the patient in a warm room and wrapping him in warm blankets may be feasible in the A&E department. Active rewarming is better done on an Intensive Care Unit where close monitoring is possible.

# *Heat stroke*

Heat stroke may be due to heat overload when heat production exceeds heat loss or due to thermoregulatory failure. The former occurs typically in sportsmen and soldiers on military training. The latter is predisposed to by the extremes of age (cf. hypothermia), dehydration, obesity, infection, alcoholism, mental illness and drug therapy which impairs heat loss.

The condition is characterized by a core temperature greater than 41°C, cerebral disturbance which ranges from confusion to coma, and warm skin which may or may not be sweating depending on the degree of dehydration.

**Pathophysiological changes of heat stroke**.    Initially the cardiac output is increased and vasodilatation occurs. Eventually the cardiac output falls. This may be due to damage to the myocardium or to dehydration as a result of profuse sweating. Urine output falls and thermal damage may cause acute tubular necrosis which can be aggravated by rhabdomyolysis.

Sodium, potassium, magnesium, calcium and phosphorus are lost in sweat. Gross electrolyte abnormalities may cause coma and muscle weakness leading to myocardial and respiratory failure. The respiratory rate increases initially and causes a respiratory alkalosis. As the problem progresses a mixed acid-base abnormality occurs due to the development of a metabolic acidosis secondary to tissue hypoxia.

The respiratory system is not directly affected by heat stroke but acidic stomach contents may be inhaled into the lungs as a result of the loss of protective airway reflexes, and prolonged tissue hypoxia may be complicated by multiple organ failure and the adult respiratory distress syndrome.

The central nervous system is damaged by hyperpyrexia in proportion to the extent and duration of the fever. Cellular dysfunction occurs in all parts of the brain and produces a variety of symptoms including convulsions and coma, both of which may be the reason for the involvement of an anaesthetist.

Thrombocytopenia and disseminated intravascular coagulation are complications of heat stroke.

**The management of heat stroke**.   As with all severely ill patients, treatment should initially be directed towards securing the airway, establishing adequate ventilation and oxygenation, and restoring the circulating blood volume. Initially physiological saline can be given but ultimately the fluid regime must be designed to include, in the correct proportions, the water and the electrolytes which are deficient. It is helpful if infusion fluids are cooled in an ice bath prior to administration. Correction of dehydration may not be sufficient to restore cardiovascular function if the myocardium is damaged and inotropic support may be necessary (Table 3.2.4, p. 186). Central venous pressure monitoring is essential and some patients may benefit from monitoring with a pulmonary artery flotation catheter, particularly if they are old or there is pre-existing heart or lung disease.

When life-saving resuscitation has commenced the patient should be cooled. This can be done by placing ice packs over major arteries and by performing stomach and bladder washouts with ice cold saline. The most effective method of cooling is to nurse the patient in the lateral position so that the greatest possible area of skin is exposed and to spray the patient with cold water while fanning him with warm air. This produces evaporation of the water and better cooling because the latent heat of evaporation of water is greater than the latent heat of warming. Whichever method is used for cooling, it is helpful to give small doses of chlorpromazine to prevent shivering which increases heat production.

Other treatment in the A&E department may include the use of anti-epileptic drugs (Table 3.3.3, p. 209) to control fits and the use of mannitol to promote a diuresis.

# *Drowning*

Victims of drowning who survive to reach the A&E department have inhaled water into the lungs. 'Dry' drowning, in contrast, results from reflex laryngospasm on entry into the water and causes rapid death due to asphyxia. Patients who have inhaled water may initially suffer a period of reflex laryngospasm, but then hypoxia and hypercarbia stimulate respiration and inhalation of water. Water is usually also swallowed and may then be vomited and inhaled into the lungs. Although there are pathophysiological distinctions between fresh and salt water drowning, the clinical presentations of both types of drowning are very similar. The patient will be cyanosed, tachypnoeic and may be coughing up pink frothy sputum. He may be agitated but alert, comatose or at any level of consciousness in between. On auscultation of the chest, rhonchi and rales may be heard. There may also be signs of head or cervical spine injury and of hypothermia.

**Pathophysiology of near-drowning.**   Inhalation of water into the lungs increases airway resistance, decreases the effectiveness of surfactant causing atelectasis, induces hypoxic pulmonary vasoconstriction and damages the alveolar capillary membrane. In fresh water drowning, water is absorbed into the circulation causing haemolysis, hyperkalaemia, haemoglobinuria and, at a later time, acute renal failure. Salt water drowning causes an efflux of water into the alveoli and pulmonary oedema. All patients are grossly hypoxic, have gross mismatch between perfusion and ventilation and decreased compliance. Infection and the adult respiratory distress syndrome may develop after 24 hours even though the patient has apparently recovered well from the initial incident. The cardiovascular system tends to be stable. Dysrhythmias secondary to hypoxia, acidosis, hyperkalaemia or hypothermia are a potential problem.

Tissue hypoxia is mainly related to the severity of the pulmonary pathology. Severe tissue hypoxia results in cerebral damage and raised intracranial pressure.

**Management of drowning**. Oxygen should be given on admission and airway, respiratory and cardiovascular insufficiency should be corrected. Bronchospasm should be treated in the same way as described for asthma (Table 3.2.2, p. 178). Controlled mechanical ventilation may be necessary if the patient is severely hypoxic or to control cerebral oedema. Severe hypoxia in spite of controlled mechanical ventilation may improve with the addition of positive end expiratory pressure. There is, however, an inevitable rise in intrathoracic pressure which may reduce venous return and increase intracranial pressure. Sometimes blood transfusion is required if haemolysis has been severe. Dysrhythmias are treated in the usual way (pp. 192–194).

# PART FOUR

# Special considerations relating to the management of paediatric accidents and emergencies

# The physiological differences between adults and children

Children are physiologically different from adults and the differences are not necessarily proportional to their size. Each child should, therefore, be treated as an individual *and should not be regarded as a scaled down adult*. Normal physiological variables for children of different ages are listed in Table 4.1. The reasons for some of these variables are discussed in the following text and examples of why they are important are given.

**Cardiovascular system**. The child's heart contains less sarcomeres and myofilaments per unit area than the adult heart

**Table 4.1 Normal physiological variables for children**

| Age (years) | Weight (kg) | Heart rate (b.p.m) | Hb (g/dl) | Respiratory rate | Urine output (ml/kg/h) |
|---|---|---|---|---|---|
| 1 | 10 | | 11.5 | | |
| 2 | 13 | 120 | 12.0 | 24+/−6 | 2 |
| 3 | 15 | | | | |
| 4 | 17 | | 12.5 | | |
| 5 | 19 | | 13.5 | 23+/−5 | 1 |
| 6 | 20 | | | | |
| 7 | 22 | 100 | | | |
| 8 | 25 | | | 20+/−6 | |
| 9 | 27 | | | | |
| 10 | 30 | 90 | 13.7 | | |
| 11 | 32 | | | | |
| 12 | 36 | | | 18+/−6 | |
| 13 | 40 | | | | |
| 14 | 45 | 85 | 14.5 | 15+/−3 | |
| 15 | 50 | | | | 0.5 |

N.B. Use as a guide only. Consensus view compiled from various sources.
Systolic BP = (2 × age) + 80.   Diastolic BP = 2/3 systolic BP.
Blood volume:   Neonate 85 ml/kg. Infant 80 ml/kg.
              Child 75 ml/kg. Adult 65–70 ml/kg.

and there are fewer mitochondria and less myosin ATPase. The immature ventricle is, therefore, non-compliant and responds poorly to volume loading. The infant depends on an increase in heart rate rather than in stoke volume to increase cardiac output. In addition the infant heart has small noradrenaline stores and insensitive beta adrenergic receptors. Infants tend to be resistant to dopamine.

Sympathetic innervation of the infant heart and blood vessels is less well developed than in the adult. The parasympathetic system is better developed although vagal tone is low. Bradycardia is a common response to hypoxia in children aged less than 5 years.

The infant's response to stress or hypovolaemia depends mainly on an increased heart rate and vasoconstriction. The blood pressure is well maintained until 20% of the blood volume is lost, when decompensation tends to occur suddenly and dramatically. The response to sepsis is similar to that seen in adults.

The child's heart does, however, have lower resting energy needs than the adult and relatively greater glycogen stores and anaerobic capacity. The infant myocardium is, therefore, more resistant to ischaemia than the adult myocardium.

Blood volume increases with age and is proportional to body weight. The smaller blood volume must be appreciated as volume losses which would be insignificant in the adult may be very important in the child. In particular, bleeding from the scalp or into the cranial cavity can cause significant hypovolaemia. So too can repeated blood sampling for haematological and biochemical investigations. Furthermore, the child's haemoglobin level is lower than in adults and hence the child's blood has less oxygen carrying capacity.

Dysrhythmias in children tend to be due to hypoxia, hypotension, raised intracranial pressure and sepsis. Several congenital heart conditions are associated with dysrhythmias.

**Respiratory system**. Respiratory function in children is related to metabolic demands and children have a lower

221

respiratory reserve than adults. Oxygen consumption in infants is 6–8 ml/kg body weight/min as opposed to 4 ml/kg/min in the adult. An increase in oxygen demand is met by an increase in respiratory rate.

The anatomy of the respiratory system has several important differences from adults. Infants are obligatory nose breathers. Nasal obstruction can be overcome by mouth breathing but the child becomes rapidly exhausted. The ribs are horizontal and bucket handle motion is minimal. The child is dependent on diaphragmatic movement for gas exchange and respiration may be severely compromised by abdominal distension. The chest wall is compliant. An increase in respiratory effort is manifest as indrawing of both the bony structures and the soft tissue. This, in combination with the greater cartilagenous content of the tracheobronchial tree, increases the tendency to airway closure, atelectasis and intrapulmonary shunting. The compliance of the chest wall can be an advantage in the case of injury. Fractured ribs are an uncommon injury.

The airways in the child are smaller than in the adult. Resistance to flow is inversely proportional to the fourth power of the radius of the airway. The child is, therefore, extremely sensitive to small changes in airway size from problems such as oedema or foreign bodies. One millimetre of oedema produces a sixteenfold increase in resistance. In addition, the cuff on an endotracheal tube significantly reduces the size of endotracheal tube which can be passed and thus increases airway resistance. Fortunately the cricoid ring in children is circular and, if a correctly sized endotracheal tube is passed, a seal can be obtained at this level without the need for a cuff.

Respiratory failure is manifest as tachypnoea and the use of the accessory muscles of respiration. In addition to flairing of the nostrils and tracheal tug, sternal and intercostal recession on inspiration are apparent. In young infants, the first signs of hypoxia may be pallor, skin blotchiness and bradycardia.

Endotracheal intubation can be difficult because the occiput is large and prevents neck extension, the tongue is large and the larynx lies at the level of C4/5 as opposed to C5 in the adult.

**Renal function**. At birth, generalized high vascular resistance and low systemic blood pressure result in a relatively low glomerular filtration rate. In addition, the glomeruli are reduced in size and number and the permeability of the basement membrane is reduced when compared to the adult. By the age of one month, however, the child's kidneys are 70% mature and are able to meet most challenges.

**Fluid, electrolyte and nutritional requirements**. The basal metabolic rate in young children is twice that of adults. When compared to adults, young children require proportionately greater amounts of water and electrolytes although this discrepancy decreases with increasing age. Children are particularly susceptible to dehydration as a result of prolonged water deprivation or excessive losses due to vomiting or diarrhoea. A 10% reduction in body water causes a decrease in conscious level, dry mucous membranes, poor skin turgor, sunken eyes and fontanelles, an increase in heart rate and respiratory rate and a decrease in urine output. A 20% reduction in body water causes coma, hypotension and oliguria or anuria. Normal water requirements are summarized in Table 4.2.

Metabolism is relatively increased in children but liver glycogen stores are small. Prolonged starvation causes hypoglycaemia.

**Table 4.2 Average paediatric maintenance intravenous fluid requirements**

| Weight | Water requirement |
|--------|-------------------|
| < 10 kg | 100 ml/kg/24 hours |
| 11–19 kg | 1000 ml plus 50 ml/kg/24 hours for each kg over 10 kg |
| > 20 kg | 1500 ml plus 20 ml / kg / 24 hours for each kg over 20 kg |

N.B. Increased requirements if the child is pyrexial or vomiting.

223

**Central nervous system**. In proportion to the size of the body, the child's brain is larger than the adult brain, being approximately 80% of the adult weight in a 2-year-old. In children up to the age of 19 months, the fontanelle is open and the dura can distend in response to an increase in intracranial volume. In the child, however, the dura is relatively non-compliant. This reduces the potential benefit of the open fontanelle as a means of maintaining normal intracranial pressure. In children, small additional volumes may cause an increase in intracranial pressure because there is relatively less space for expansion than there is in the adult skull. A rise in pressure, therefore, occurs earlier than in the adult because the compliance of the dura is relatively less and the cranial cavity is smaller. The speed of the rise in pressure, after the critical volume has been reached, is slower. Cerebral blood flow is lower in the child than the adult and autoregulation of cerebral blood flow is thought to occur at lower pressures than in the adult but precise values are not known. This means that the child ought to tolerate mild hypotension better than the adult. In practice, children do appear to recover better than adults from cerebral insults although it appears that hypoxia is equally damaging at any age. In the child, the cerebral vasculature is thought to be less responsive to hypocarbia than in the adult.

In children, assessment of the depth of coma can be difficult because the ability to vocalize may be limited by immaturity. Examples of systems for scoring the verbal component of the Glasgow Coma Scale are shown in Table 4.3. The systems tend to be less easy to interpret than the adult equivalent and it can be helpful if the same person is responsible for repeated assessments.

The child is particularly susceptible to fits. These occur commonly following head injury, during hypoxic and hypoglycaemic episodes and during febrile illnesses. They result in increased cerebral oxygen demand and must be treated either with anti-epileptic drugs or by correcting the underlying cause.

Children experience pain in the same way as adults. Not only does the pain make the child difficult to handle in the

224

**Table 4.3 Glasgow Coma Score: scoring the verbal response in children**

| Score | Pons[1] | Adelaide[2] | ATLS[3] |
|-------|---------|-------------|---------|
| 5 | Orientated | Orientated | Appropriate words, social smile, fixes and follows |
| 4 | Confused | Says words | Cries but consolable |
| 3 | Inappropriate words | Vocal sounds | Persistently irritable |
| 2 | Garbled words | Cries | Restless, agitated |
| 1 | None | None | None |

1. Pons, P.T. (1990). Head trauma. In *Emergency Pediatrics: a Guide to Ambulatory Care* (R.M. Barkin, ed.), 3rd edn. St Louis: C.V. Mosby Co., pp 337–347.
2. Simpson, D. and Reilly, P. (1982). Paediatric coma scale. *Lancet*, **ii**, 450.
3. American College of Surgeons. (1989). *Advanced Trauma Life Support Course Manual.* Chicago: American College of Surgeons.

A&E department, but it also may affect the child's attitude to illness and hospitals in general. Most of the techniques used for adults are suitable for children provided that drugs are administered in suitable paediatric doses.

Children are particularly susceptible to stress and anxiety. Sedation can be provided by administering morphine 0.05 mg/kg intravenously and midazolam 0.05 mg/kg. These should be administered with caution with the same provisos that apply to adults (pp. 80–82).

**Temperature control**.   Children have a large surface area in relation to their weight and are thus susceptible to heat loss. The head is large in proportion to the rest of the body and a significant amount of heat can be lost from this area. Thermoregulation in children is not as well developed as in adults. Children can easily become hypothermic. This is a particular problem in A&E departments where clothing must be removed in order that the child may be properly examined and treated and where the ambient temperature can be less than in other areas of the hospital.

**Table 4.4 Paediatric drug doses**

General anaesthetic agents
| | |
|---|---|
| Etomidate | not recommended |
| Ketamine | 2 mg/kg IV, 10 mg/kg IM |
| Propofol | 2–2.5mg/kg IV |
| Thiopentone | 4 mg/kg IV |
| Suxamethonium | 1 mg/kg IV |
| Alcuronium | 0.2 mg/kg IV |
| Atracurium | 0.3–0.6 mg/kg IV |
| d-tubocurine | 0.3–0.5 mg/kg IV |
| Pancuronium | 0.06–0.1 mg/kg IV |
| Vecuronium | 0.08–0.1 mg/kg IV |
| Atropine | 0.02 mg/kg IV |

Local anaesthetics
| | |
|---|---|
| Bupivacaine | maximum dose 2 mg/kg |
| Lignocaine | maximum dose 3 mg/kg; 7 mg/kg with adrenaline |
| Prilocaine | maximum dose 6 mg/kg; 8 mg/kg with adrenaline |

Analgesics
| | |
|---|---|
| Alfentanyl | 0.03–0.05 mg/kg IV |
| Codeine phosphate | 0.5 mg/kg IM |
| Fentanyl | 0.015 mg/kg IV |
| Morphine | 0.2 mg/kg IM, 0.1 mg/kg IV |
| Papaveretum | 0.3 mg/kg IM, 0.15 mg/kg IM |
| Pethidine | 2 mg/kg IM, 1 mg/kg IV |

Sedatives and anti-epileptic drugs
| | |
|---|---|
| Chlormethiazole | 0.08 mg/kg/min IV |
| Diazepam | 0.1 mg/kg IV |
| Midazolam | 0.05 mg/kg IV |
| Phenytoin | 10–20 mg/kg IV |
| Paraldehyde | 150 mg/kg IM |

Drugs acting on the cardiovascular system
| | |
|---|---|
| Adrenaline (1:1000) | 0.01 ml/kg IV |
| Atropine | 0.01–0.02 mg/kg IV |
| Bretylium | 5 mg/kg |
| Calcium chloride | 20–30 mg/kg |
| Digitalis | 0.02 mg/kg IV |
| Dobutamine | 1–15 µg/kg IV |
| Dopamine | 2–20 µg/kg IV |
| Glucagon | 0.03–0.1 mg/kg IV |
| Isoprenaline | 0.05–1.5 µg/kg IV |
| Labetolol | 0.5–1.0 mg/kg IV |
| Lignocaine | 1 mg/kg IV |

| | |
|---|---|
| Nitroglycerin | not recommended |
| Noradrenaline | 0.1–1.0 µg/kg/min IV |
| Procainamide | 2–6 mg/kg IV |
| Salbutamol | 5 µg/kg IV |
| Sodium nitroprusside | 0.5–10 µg/kg/min IV |
| | |
| Diuretics | |
| Frusemide | 1 mg/kg IV |
| Mannitol | 500 mg/kg IV |
| | |
| Drugs acting on the respiratory tract | |
| Aminophylline | 6 mg/kg IV |
| Ipratropium bromide | 100–500 µg nebulized |
| Salbutamol | 2.5 mg nebulized |
| Terbutaline | 0.01 mg/kg SC |
| | |
| Miscellaneous | |
| Dicobalt edetate | 4 mg/kg IV |
| Flumazenil | dose not yet decided ? 3 µg/kg IV |
| Naloxone | 5 µg/kg IV |
| Pralidoxime | 20–50 mg/kg IV |
| Sodium nitrite | ⎫ Consult Poisons Information Centre. |
| Sodium thiosulphate | ⎬ Telephone numbers in British National |
| | ⎭ Formulary. |

**Response to drugs**. Due to the immaturity of children's organs, the response to drugs is often different from that of adults. Furthermore, the relatively larger cardiac output may affect the distribution and action of drugs. Paediatric drug doses are summarized in Table 4.4. Most drugs are supplied in doses and volumes suitable for adults which means that the correct paediatric dose is contained in a ridiculously small volume which may be impossible to measure accurately. It is important that drugs are administered accurately and that the dose is carefully calculated on the basis of the patient's weight. If necessary, the drug should be diluted up to a more suitable volume. It is imperative that intravenous cannulae are flushed in order to ensure that the drug reaches the circulation and equally important that the volume of drug and flush solution is included in fluid balance calculations.

**Summary**. The following guidelines may be helpful:

1. The normal response to hypovolaemia and myocardial insufficiency is tachycardia.
2. The child has a small blood volume and immature cardiovascular system. Dehydration and small blood losses can cause significant haemodynamic changes.
3. Decompensation due to cardiovascular insufficiency may be sudden and catastrophic.
4. Due to the child's high metabolic rate, oxygen consumption is high. Increased oxygen demand is met by an increase in respiratory rate. Airway narrowing dramatically increases the resistance to gas flow and even minor obstructions can cause significant respiratory distress.
5. Intracranial pressure may be increased by small increases in the volume of intracranial contents.
6. Pain is felt by children and must be controlled.
7. Hypoglycaemia and dehydration may be precipitated by relatively short periods of fluid and food deprivation.
8. Hypothermia is an ever present problem.
9. Drug doses must be meticulously calculated, drawn up and administered.

**FURTHER READING**

Kahana, M.D. (1990). Acute pain management in children: neural blockade and patient controlled analgesia. In *Anesthetic Management of Difficult and Routine Pediatric Patients*, 2nd edn (Berry, F.A., ed.). New York: Churchill-Livingstone, pp. 323–340.

# The response to injury and illness

The response of children to illness and injury may be 'abnormal' to their adult doctors but these so-called abnormalities may be a valuable aid to diagnosis. The physiological differences in response to illness and injury have been discussed in the previous section. Other differences, which are often subtle and difficult to quantify, are also important.

Normally a distressed child will cry or scream and will become red in the face. The quiet, pale child may be too ill to cry, may have a reduced conscious level or may be severely anaemic and/or hypovolaemic. The child may also be quiet because abdominal or chest pain is aggravated by crying. Inability or unwillingness to communicate may also be one of the first clues that child abuse has occurred. Interpretation of an existing cry may also be helpful. A persistent cry in an apparently normal child may indicate occult illness or injury. A high pitched cry usually indicates cerebral irritation or raised intracranial pressure.

Drowsiness, floppiness or respiratory distress may all be non-specific signs of severe illness or injury.

Vomiting is a common response to injury and illness. In the the head injured child, it does not necessarily indicate raised intracranial pressure unless it is persistent.

Thirst may be a manifestation of dehydration but is also a useful early sign of hypovolaemia caused by blood or plasma loss.

Attention should always be given to the history of the injury which is given by relatives or carers. If accurate, it may give valuable clues to the diagnosis. Coughing during eating, for example, may be a clue that the cause of respiratory distress is due to the inhalation of a foreign body. The history may, however, not be accurate. Injuries which do not appear to be compatible with the supposed cause may be non-accidental. Another clue to non-accidental injury is the presence of old injuries on X-rays. Children are known to suffer Munchausen's syndrome by proxy.

As in adults, it is vital that there is a protocol for the management of children. This is similar to that used in adults:

1. On admission, the child should be assessed for airway, breathing and cardiovascular insufficiency (primary sur-

vey). Appropriate life-saving resuscitation should be commenced promptly.

2. When life-saving resuscitation is in progress and the immediate threat to life has been removed, a history should, if possible, be obtained from ambulance staff or relatives. All clothes should be removed. The child should then be examined from head to toe (secondary survey) and appropriate investigations performed. As soon as the examination is complete the child should be covered with a warm blanket to prevent further heat loss.

3. The examination and investigations should enable a provisional diagnosis to be made and definitive treatment and monitoring to be started.

4. Ideally the child should then be transferred to a paediatric ward. If the child is not stable enough for transfer, the results of treatment should be assessed and inappropriate responses identified.

5. The cause of an inappropriate response should be sought. It may be due to inadequate or inappropriate treatment of a correctly diagnosed condition or due to failure to make the correct diagnosis and therefore failure to administer the correct treatment.

# Respiratory tract obstruction

**The causes and pathophysiology of respiratory tract obstruction**. Airway obstruction may be extrathoracic or intrathoracic. The causes of airway obstruction are classified in Table 4.5. As has already been described, the small diameter of the child's airways means that even a small decrease in airway diameter can cause a dramatic increase in resistance to breathing. Extrathoracic obstruction causes inspiratory stridor. Intrathoracic obstruction causes expiratory wheeze and air trapping. Retraction of the chest wall permits excessive negative intrathoracic pressures to be generated which may be transmitted to the lung and result in pulmonary oedema.

**Table 4.5 Causes of respiratory insufficiency in children**

| | |
|---|---|
| 1. Upper airway obstruction | (a) swelling<br>    i. thermal<br>    ii. allergy<br>    iii. infection<br>(b) foreign body<br>(c) tumour<br>(d) loss of protective airway reflexes<br>    i. head injury<br>    ii. hypoxia/hypovolaemia<br>    iii. drugs/alcohol<br>    iv. metabolic/endocrine<br>(e) laryngeal trauma |
| 2. Inadequate chest wall and diaphragmatic excursion | (a) trauma (Table 1.2.1, p. 36)<br>(b) pleuritic pain<br>(c) neurological disorders<br>(d) burns (Table 2.2.3, p. 135)<br>(e) abdominal pain and swelling |
| 3. Inadequate lung expansion | (a) inadequate chest wall excursion<br>(b) trauma (Table 1.2.1, p. 36)<br>(c) burns (Table 2.2.3, p. 135)<br>(d) spontaneous pneumothorax<br>(e) pleural effusion<br>(f) infective consolidation<br>(g) pulmonary collapse due to a sputum plug or foreign body<br>(h) bronchospasm |
| 4. Inadequate respiratory drive | (a) coma (Table 3.2.5, p. 188)<br>(b) head injury<br>(c) hypoxia/hypovolaemia<br>(d) poisoning<br>(e) metabolic |
| 5. Impaired gas exchange | (a) trauma (Table 1.2.1, p. 36)<br>(b) burns (Table 2.2.3, p. 135)<br>(c) pulmonary collapse<br>(d) pulmonary consolidation<br>(e) pulmonary aspiration of stomach contents<br>(f) pulmonary embolism<br>(g) inadequate pulmonary perfusion |

Hypocarbia is a common finding due to the increased respiratory rate. Hypoxia usually develops late, although this depends on the aetiology of the obstruction.

**Clinical signs of airway obstruction**. A history of sudden choking and difficulty in breathing during eating or play is a clue that airway obstruction may be due to a foreign body. Stridor is the cardinal sign of extrathoracic airway obstruction. Voice sounds may also be helpful as they alter depending on the level of the obstruction. Supraglottic obstructions muffle the voice whereas glottic obstructions cause harsh voice sounds or aphonia. As with adults, excessive salivation and drooling is common with supraglottic obstruction.

Retraction of the chest wall and use of the accessory muscles of respiration are evidence of the difficulty being experienced with breathing past the obstruction.

Auscultation will identify inspiratory stridor or expiratory wheeze, but there may be difficulty distinguishing between the two just as there is in adults (pp. 129–131).

Pyrexia gives clues to an infective aetiology such as epiglottitis, croup or tonsillitis.

**General management of airway obstruction**. In general, if the child is in extremis, oxygen should be given, the airway secured and ventilation established. The methods described for adults are appropriate but a nasopharyngeal airway or nasotracheal intubation under anaesthesia is often preferred for children because plump, flabby cheeks make it more difficult to ensure that the endotracheal tube is securely fixed. Caution should be exercised before endotracheal intubation is attempted as instrumentation of a swollen epiglottis may aggravate oedema and cause total obstruction.

If intubation fails, surgical cricothyroidotomy is relatively contraindicated in children aged less than 10 years. This is because the cricoid ring is the only completely rigid part of the upper respiratory tract and inadvertent damage to the posterior part of the ring may cause tracheal collapse. Needle cricothyroidotomy is acceptable.

# SPECIFIC AIRWAY OBSTRUCTIONS

**Epiglottitis**. The onset of epiglottitis is usually acute and consists of high fever, toxaemia and noisy breathing. Epiglottitis is usually caused by *Haemophilus influenzae* and commonly affects children aged between 2 and 5 years. It can, however, occur at any age and even in adults. The child sits upright, breathes with the mouth open and has difficulty swallowing saliva. Stridor is present but is often accompanied by an expiratory snore. Because of the risk of sudden respiratory obstruction, the child is best left undisturbed, breathing oxygen through a face mask, although the diagnosis could be confirmed by soft tissue X-rays of the neck. Endotracheal intubation is ideally performed in the operating theatre with the surgeon standing by so that an emergency tracheostomy may be performed if endotracheal intubation is impossible. Prompt commencement of intravenous cefuroxime, 25 mg/kg body weight four times daily, is helpful as it will assist with rapid resolution of the epiglottic infection and swelling.

**Laryngotracheobronchitis (Croup)**. Croup is sometimes mistaken for epiglottitis and vice versa. The differences are summarized in Table 4.6. It is nearly always caused by *para-influenza* viruses although sometimes it has an allergic causation. It is rare in children under 6 months of age and commonly affects the 6-months to 2-year-old age group. The clinical onset may follow a prodromal upper respiratory tract infection and consists of a low grade fever, harsh barking cough and hoarse voice. The onset is usually less acute than that of epiglottitis and chest retraction and the use of the accessory muscles of respiration are a late sign. Auscultation reveals an expiratory wheeze which is due in part to airway oedema and in part due to obstruction of the bronchi by infected secretions.

Oxygen should be given. Airway obstruction may be relieved by nebulization of racemic adrenaline. The usual dose is 0.5 ml/kg body weight of standard 1:1000 adrenaline, diluted if necessary, to produce a volume of 2 ml. In the

**Table 4.6 The differential diagnosis of epiglottitis and croup**

|  | Epiglottitis | Croup |
|---|---|---|
| Age (common) | 2–5 years | 6 months–2 years |
| Age (range) | 1 year–adult | Up to 5 years |
| Preceding respiratory infection | Rare | Usual |
| Onset | Hours | Days |
| Obstruction | Supraglottic oedema | Subglottic oedema and secretions |
| Fever | High | Low grade |
| Preferred posture | Sitting | Variable |
| Drooling | Marked | Minimal |
| Dysphagia | Marked | None |
| Voice | Clear/muffled | Hoarse |
| Stridor | Inspiratory | Inspiratory/expiratory |
| Cough | None | Barking |
| Sore throat | Common | Rare |

presence of hypoxia unrelieved by oxygen through a face mask, increasing tachypnoea and signs of respiratory distress, endotracheal intubation is indicated. The tube size used should be have an internal diameter of at least 1 mm less than that predicted by the patient's age. Dexamethasone is thought to improve the rate of recovery.

**Acute tonsillar enlargement.** This often occurs as a result of acute infection and the clinical signs may mimic epiglottitis. Management is by relief of airway obstruction with a nasopharyngeal airway or nasotracheal tube. Tonsillectomy is usually contraindicated during acute infection because bleeding is increased. *Retropharyngeal abscess, peritonsillar abscess, infectious mononucleosis* and *Ludwig's angina* may produce similar symptoms and may also mimic epiglottitis. Control of the airway is vital. Drainage and antibiotic therapy may also be indicated.

**Subglottic haemangioma.** These lesions may cause airway obstruction in the second and third months of life. Cutaneous lesions often provide a clue to the diagnosis. Endotracheal intubation may precipitate torrential bleeding and be life threatening due to lower airway obstruction by blood and, possibly, hypovolaemia. If the diagnosis is suspected, it should be confirmed at bronchoscopy and the airway obstruction relieved by a formal tracheostomy.

**Foreign body**. Inhaled foreign bodies are a common problem in infants aged between 6 months and 2 years of age. They should be suspected if the obstruction is acute and occurs during eating or playing. Pharyngeal impaction usually causes gagging, respiratory distress and facial congestion. Laryngeal impaction causes stridor, cough and aphonia. Tracheal or bronchial foreign bodies cause persistent coughing and wheeze. Large foreign bodies impacted in the oesophagus may cause obstruction of the relevant part of the airway.

Foreign bodies in the pharynx or larynx may be dislodged by placing the child prone in a head down position. Several backblows between the shoulder blades may dislodge the foreign body. The Heimlich manoeuvre is not recommended because intra-abdominal organs may be damaged. If backblows fail, chest thrusts or a finger sweep across the pharynx may work although the latter may impact the foreign body in the larynx. The best method of removal is achieved under direct vision using a laryngoscope or bronchoscope and forceps.

**Asthma**. The clinical presentation of asthma is very similar in children to that in adults although chest recession may be more obvious. Treatment principles are the same (pp. 203–206) although the doses of drugs are reduced (Table 4.4, p. 227).

**Bronchiolitis**. Bronchiolitis usually occurs in children aged less than 6 months. It causes a cough, low grade fever, tachypnoea and wheeze due to small airways oedema and infected secretions. It is usually caused by the *respiratory syncytial* virus. Treatment consists of oxygen via a face mask and attention to fluid balance. Severe cases benefit from nasopharyngeal or nasotracheal continuous airways pressure.

# Acute respiratory insufficiency

The causes of acute respiratory insufficiency in children are listed in Table 4.5 and are classified in a similar manner to adults. The only difference is that inadequate or inappropriate movement of the chest wall includes conditions causing inadequate or inappropriate movement of the diaphragm. This is because the child depends on adequate excursion of the diaphragm for gas exchange rather than movement of the rib cage. It is, however, important to bear in mind that as the child grows older the contribution of the chest wall to ventilation becomes increasingly more important. As this happens the ribs move from the horizontal to the adult position. The appearance of the ribs on the chest X-ray can be used as a guide to the likely importance of chest wall movement.

Some of the signs of respiratory insufficiency have been described on p. 232. Auscultation reveals the same sounds as in adults and the interpretation of auscultatory findings is the same.

Most of the causes of respiratory insufficiency are the same as in adults. There are two exceptions.

**Acute respiratory failure secondary to heart disease**.   In the adult, respiratory failure secondary to heart disease is usually related to acquired myocardial lesions such as rheumatic valve disease or ischaemic heart disease. In the child, respiratory failure is usually secondary to congenital heart conditions. There are three major causes. First, left ventricular failure and pulmonary oedema occur because blood flow from the left ventricle is obstructed. This can be due to coarctation of the aorta or aortic stenosis. Second, pulmonary oedema can occur because of large left to right shunts which overload the left ventricle. A patent ductus arteriosus and ventricular septal defects cause this type of problem. Third, abnormalities of pulmonary blood flow such as that occurring in Fallot's tetralogy, transposition of the great vessels or with a single ventricle result in incomplete oxygenation of the blood and systemic arterial hypoxia.

All infants with severe congenital heart disease are at risk of developing intercurrent pulmonary infections which, in combination with existing pulmonary abnormalities, may precipitate acute respiratory insufficiency.

**Trauma**.   Injury to the ribs is less common in children than in adults but major intrathoracic injuries such as haemothorax, pneumothorax, pulmonary contusion and rupture of the diaphragm often occur in the absence of fractured ribs.

All injuries, including minor ones such as Colles fracture, completely inhibit or delay stomach emptying. Gastric dilatation increases the volume of the abdominal contents and may splint the diaphragm. Similar problems occur if the child is unable to pass urine and the bladder becomes distended.

**Inhalation of gastric contents**.   This is a risk in children with obtunded airway reflexes due to hypoxia, hypovolaemia, injury or severe illness. In young children the bronchi lie at equal angles to the trachea and aspirated stomach contents pass into the right and left lungs with equal frequency. The pathophysiological results of the pulmonary inhalation of stomach contents are the same as in adults (pp. 102–103).

The management principles of acute respiratory insufficiency are similar to those for adults. The problems are mainly practical. Oxygen masks, for example, are not well tolerated by young children and it may be more appropriate to nurse the child in an oxygen tent. Many of these tents are incapable of delivering more than 40% oxygen and the concentration is further reduced every time the tent is opened. If adequate oxygenation cannot be maintained, endotracheal intubation and controlled mechanical ventilation are indicated.

# Hypovolaemia

In children, the response to hypovolaemia is an increase in heart rate and vasoconstriction. Frank hypotension occurs when more than 40% of the blood volume has been lost. At this stage, urgent resuscitation is essential. Ideally, resuscitation should be commenced at the first signs of hypovolaemia when approximately 25% of the blood volume has been lost. At this stage, the pulse will have become weak and thready, the child will be lethargic, irritable or confused, the skin is cool and clammy and the urine output is reduced. Initially, resuscitation can be started with a challenge of crystalloid fluid in a dose of 20 ml/kg body weight. This can be repeated three times. If the reponse is inadequate, the fluid used should be changed to a colloid. Significant red cell loss must be replaced with blood as soon as it is available. In the presence of persistent hypotension due to blood loss, group O-negative or type-specific blood must be given if fully crossmatched blood is not available.

Venous access can be difficult to obtain in children particularly in toddlers who tend to be chubby. Central veins can be used, as can a venous cut down. In children less than 6 years of age, interosseous transfusion through the anterior tibial plateau or the distal end of the femur can provide a rapid method of access. The circulation time to the heart is about 20 seconds and drugs as well as fluids can be given by this route. The only exception is bretylium. Interosseous transfusion cannulae can be purchased but if one is not available a bone marrow aspiration needle can be used.

# Cardiac arrest

In principle, the diagnosis, causes and management of cardiac arrest in children is similar to adults. The differences are due to the different size and weight of children. The management of cardiac arrest is summarized in Tables 4.7, 4.8 and 4.9.

## FURTHER READING

Zideman, D.A. (1986). Resuscitation of infants and children. *Br. Med. J.,* **292**, 1584–1588.

# *Loss of consciousness*

Loss of consciousness in the child has similar causes to those listed for adults (Table 3.2.5, p. 188). Initially management is directed towards maintaining a clear airway, ensuring adequate ventilation and restoring circulating blood volume. Children are sensitive to hypoxia and hypovolaemia and manual support of the airway and the administration of oxygen and a fluid challenge are often sufficient to restore consciousness very quickly. Similarly, hypoglycaemia and

**Table 4.7 Basic paediatric life support**

|  | *Baby* | *Child* | *Adult* |
|---|---|---|---|
| External chest compressions (per min) | 120 | 100 | 60 |
| Depth of chest compressions (cm) | 1–1.5 | 2–3 | 4–5 |
| Rate of ventilation (per min) | 24 | 20 | 12 |

d.c. shock dose = 2 joules/kg

Internal diameter of uncuffed endotracheal tube (mm) = (age/4) + 4.5
Rough guide to endotracheal tube size = size of child's little finger

N.B. Precordial blow prior to external cardiac massage not recommended for children.

**Table 4.8 Protocol for paediatric cardiac arrest**

| *External cardiac massage* | PLUS | *Oxygen* | PLUS | *Controlled mechanical ventilation* |
|---|---|---|---|---|
| Asystole | | Ventricular Fibrillation | | Electromechanical dissociation |
| ↓ | | ↓ | | ↓ |
| Adrenaline 0.1 ml/kg (1:10 000) | | d.c. shock 1–2 joules/kg | | Adrenaline 0.1 ml/kg (1:10 000) |
| ↓ | | ↓ | | ↓ |
| Atropine 0.02 mg/kg | | d.c. shock 2 joules/kg | | Physiological saline 20 ml/kg |
| ↓ | | ↓ | | ↓ |
| Repeat adrenaline | | Lignocaine 1 mg/kg | | Consider Cardiac tamponade Tension pneumothorax |
| ↓ | | ↓ | | |
| Repeat atropine | | d.c. Shock 2 joules/kg | | |
| ↓ | | ↓ | | |
| Repeat adrenaline | | Adrenaline 0.1 ml/kg (1:10 000) | | |
| | | ↓ | | |
| | | d.c. shock 2 joules/kg | | |
| | | ↓ | | |
| | | Bretylium 5–10 mg/kg | | |
| | | ↓ | | |
| | | d.c. shock 2 joules/kg | | |

hyperglycaemia can be rapidly treated. If recovery of consciousness is likely to be rapid, it is unnecessary to place an endotracheal tube in the child. If there is any doubt, however, and the risk of vomiting and pulmonary inhalation of gastric contents is great, it is better to intubate the child and to remove the endotracheal tube as soon as consciousness returns.

**Table 4.9 Paediatric dose table for cardiac arrest**

| | | | | | | |
|---|---|---|---|---|---|---|
| Age (years) | 1 | 3 | 6 | 10 | 13 | 15 |
| Weight (kg) | 10 | 15 | 20 | 30 | 40 | 50 |
| Adrenaline (1:10 000) | 1 | 1.5 | 2 | 3 | 4 | 5 |
| Atropine (0.6 mg/ml) | 0.3 | 0.45 | 0.65 | 1.0 | 1.0 | 1.0 |
| Lignocaine 1% (10 mg/ml) | 1 | 1.5 | 2 | 3 | 4 | 5 |
| Bretylium (100 mg/2 ml) | 1 | 1.5 | 2 | 3 | 4 | 5 |
| Glucose 50% | 20 | 30 | 40 | 60 | 80 | 100 |
| Sodium bicarbonate 8.4% | 10 | 15 | 20 | 30 | 40 | 50 |

N.B. Doses given in millilitres

# *Other problems*

As has already been stressed, the child should not be regarded as a small adult. In spite of this, with the exceptions already described, the *principles of management* are very similar. The physiological and size differences between adults and children should always be remembered. If this is done, the A&E anaesthetist should be able to initiate life-saving therapy, even if specialist paediatric advice is not immediately available.

# PART FIVE

# Life-threatening problems for the anaesthetist in the emergency room: the last word

# *The last word*

*Always remember: hypoxia, hypovolaemia and myocardial insufficiency will, alone or in combination, cause tissue hypoxia.*

# *Tissue hypoxia causes cellular dysfunction and death*

Anaesthetists are trained in the recognition and management of airway, breathing and circulatory problems. So are other members of the Accident and Emergency department staff. *A well organized team approach to the management of airway breathing and circulatory problems will save lives.* This is true no matter whether the patient is the victim of an accident, fire or medical or surgical emergency.

# Index

245

# Index

# Index

# Index

# Index

# Index

# Index